SACRED PATHS

SACRED PATHS

Essays on Wisdom, Love, and Mystical Realization

GEORG FEUERSTEIN

PUBLISHED FOR THE PAUL BRUNTON
PHILOSOPHIC FOUNDATION BY

LARSON PUBLICATIONS

International Standard Book Number: 0–943914–56–6
Library of Congress Catalog Card Number: 91–62548

Manufactured in the United States of America

Published for the
Paul Brunton Philosophic Foundation
by Larson Publications
4936 State Route 414
Burdett, NY 14818 USA

98 97 96 95 94 93 92 91

10 9 8 7 6 5 4 3 2 1

Grateful acknowledgment is made to J.P. Tarcher Inc., Los Angeles, for permission
to print the essay "Immortality and Freedom: India's Perspective" from the
anthology *What Survives?* by Gary Doore, 1990.

Author and publisher wish to thank the following persons and organizations for
the courtesy to reproduce their art: Photos of Sri Ramakrishna and Swami
Vivekananda by permission of the Ramakrishna-Vivekananda Center, New York;
photo of Paramahansa Yogananda by permission of the Self-Realization Fellowship,
Los Angeles; photo of Paul Brunton by permission of the Paul Brunton Philosophic
Foundation, Burdett, New York; drawings of flute-playing Krishna and Shankara by
permission of Lydia dePole, Cobb, California; photos of Theos Bernard by
permission of Eleanore Murray, Calimesa, California; photo of Lee Sannella by
permission of Lee Sanella; drawing of serpent and egg by permission of
Steven Royster, Rock Creek, Ohio.

Book & cover design/production: Paperwork, Ithaca, New York

For Greg, with my love and gratitude,
for providing the right kind of circumstance

CONTENTS

FOREWORD

When I first became enamored of Indian philosophy back in the mid-sixties, there were precious few popular books available on the subject. So, quite naturally for a student at a university renowned for its Asian studies department, I turned to scholarly literature. What I found, with some notable exceptions, were either dry academic discussions of esoteric doctrines, often translated from the German, or flowery Victorian translations of classic texts that frequently obscured the truths they purported to reveal.

Later, when my interest turned to the practice of yoga, I came across a few how-to books filled with black-and-white photographs of Indian adepts in contorted postures, but nothing that gave a broad overview of both philosophy and practice.

In the 1970s, when our collective love affair with things Eastern reached its peak, yoga books proliferated, and every swami, guru, and self-appointed adept hurried to put forward his or her own partial view of the vast panorama of yoga (which, as the author of this volume makes clear, includes far more than hatha yoga). Unfortunately, these books, although fascinating and often quite informative, were generally restricted in scope by the sectarian biases of a particular lineage or school and by the author's limited knowledge of the historical literature.

Meanwhile, scholars were taking a renewed interest in the yoga tradition, but their books, encumbered by footnotes and esoteric terminology, seemed for the most part to fall into the classic academic trap of describing abstractly and from afar what is in fact the most immediate of experiences, the evolution of spiritual awareness.

In the last decade, Sanskrit scholar Georg Feuerstein has made a unique and inestimable contribution to the yoga literature in English by combining impeccable scholarship with the immediacy of one who has practiced yoga himself. In books like *Yoga: The Technology of Ecstasy* and *The Encyclopedic Dictionary of Yoga,* he has for the first time made the entire three-thousand-year-old tradition available to the casual reader, plainly and comprehensively, yet without sacrificing the depth and subtlety that are so intrinsic to yoga.

Indeed, Feuerstein is that rarity among religious scholars—one who has deeply experienced the subject matter he teaches. Rather than pursuing academic advancement, he has, over the years, pursued his own spiritual development. The result has been an outpouring of popular books on yoga and vedanta that speak to our hearts and our spiritual aspirations as well as to our bodies and minds.

In Feuerstein's writings, the truth is a living presence; although he makes no claims to being a guru, the essays in *Sacred Paths* are not merely *about* yoga (or vedanta or tantra), they teach the essence of these philosophies with genuine passion and authority, but without sectarian bias. Take, for example, the chapter entitled "Talking with Pantanjali," in which the author has fashioned an inspiring, at times humorous, and, of course, thoroughly imaginary conversation with this great sage. Only Feuerstein—scholar, practitioner, and, dare I say it, something of a sage himself—could have pulled it off.

Like the more exhaustive *Yoga: The Technology of Ecstasy, Sacred Paths* covers a broad range of practices and teachings, from meditation and purification to sacramental sexuality, with a lucidity that will appeal to newcomers, and an erudition that will delight the most advanced of readers. Yet here we also have Feuerstein the independent thinker and commentator, weaving his own insights and interpretations into the fabric of timeless yoga wisdom. The blend is inspiring, provocative—and a pleasure to read. Yoga comes alive in these pages as a multifaceted teaching with an illustrious history that also has immediate relevance for our lives.

Begin this book casually, if you choose; read a chapter here or there as the impulse arises. But be prepared to find yourself returning to it again and again as an enduring source of spiritual and intellectual sustenance. There is no book on the yoga tradition that I can recommend more highly than this one.

STEPHAN BODIAN
Editor, *Yoga Journal*
Berkeley, California
June 1991

PREFACE

To restore the sacred to our lives has become a foremost imperative. We cannot hope to recover our personal wholeness without also rediscovering the dimension of the holy, however we may choose to conceive it. The ideology of scientism, which governs Western thought and culture and is increasingly influential throughout the world, has succeeded in obscuring that most fundamental dimension of existence. However, the sacred is merely buried, not totally annihilated. In our endeavor to rediscover it, we would do well to draw from the fountain of wisdom present in all the great spiritual traditions of humankind.

This book focuses on three of these magnificent traditions—Yoga, Vedanta, and Tantra. They are among India's finest contributions to our modern struggle for self-definition and spiritual renewal. All have a long history; all have evolved under the guiding influence of some of humanity's finest seers and sages.

Sacred Paths consists of twenty-six essays exploring different aspects of Yoga, Vedanta, and Tantra, as well as their relevance for the Western world. Nearly half of the essays are new. The others first appeared, in some instances almost two decades ago, in such magazines as *Yoga Journal, Yoga Today, Yoga and Health,* and *Clarion Call.* I have revised all of them, and in many cases have added material—in some cases substantial amounts—to round out or clarify the consideration.

I have arranged the essays in such a way that they can profitably be read in sequence. However, it should be borne in mind that they are not interwoven chapters but self-contained, if related, writings. I believe that, together, they can serve as a reliable and readable introduction to Hindu spirituality.

But this volume is not only for beginners. More advanced students will likewise find illuminating discussions in it and perhaps even some novelties, such as my treatment of the little known school of *taraka-yoga*. Furthermore, the present volume complements my other books on the subject, including my comprehensive study of Yoga entitled *Yoga: The Technology of Ecstasy*.

I am very grateful to Larson Publications for releasing this volume so efficiently and so quickly, and especially to the editor, Paul Cash, for his warm enthusiasm and judicious and sensitive editing. My wife, Trisha, has, as usual, perused everything and eliminated a number of errors and other shortcomings from the manuscript. Her passionate interest in animal rights and animal welfare has greatly sensitized me to the important issues involved, and this is reflected in some of the later essays. To her go my special gratitude and love.

GEORG FEUERSTEIN
Lake County
Northern California

1

WHAT IS YOGA?

In the West, Yoga is widely practiced as a form of calisthenics or fitness training. The headstand has become a symbol of this approach. For the outsider, this posture (*asana*) looks intriguing and difficult to do. In fact, it is comparatively easy to learn, and there are far more difficult postures that require many months of daily practice and sometimes years before they are fully mastered.

But the postures are only the "skin" of Yoga. Hidden behind them are the "flesh and blood" of breath control and mental techniques that are still more difficult to learn, as well as moral practices that require a lifetime of dedicated application. Then, corresponding to the skeletal structure of the body, there are the higher practices of ecstasy (*samadhi*) in which the ordinary mind and sensory functioning are transcended.

At the core of Yoga is the realization of the transcendental Reality itself, however it may be conceived. This aspect is not at all obvious when we watch someone perform complicated postures with great elegance. To be sure, many Western (and Eastern) practitioners are themselves not particularly aware of that spiritual dimension of Yoga. Without it, however, Yoga remains on the level of a pastime. The traditional purpose of Yoga has always been to bring about a profound transformation in the person through the transcendence of the ego. It is therefore good to remind ourselves of the meaning of Yoga.

Yoga is not easy to define. In most general terms, the Sanskrit word *yoga* stands for "spiritual discipline" in Hinduism and also in certain schools of Buddhism. A spiritual practitioner is known as a *yogin* (if male) or a *yogini* (if female).[1] More specifically, Yoga is a particular branch on the huge tree of Hindu spirituality.

As I have shown in my book *Yoga: The Technology of Ecstasy*, the roots of Yoga reach back into the ancient past.[2] Arising from archaic Shamanism, Yoga developed into an immensely complex tradition with rather fuzzy edges, which makes it difficult at times to demarcate it from the other branches of Hindu spirituality.

In its earliest identifiable form, Yoga was connected with the sacrificial ritualism of the Vedic tribes who invaded northern India some 3,500 years ago. Vedic Yoga consisted primarily in techniques of mental concentration, breath control, and chanting, which all served the religious ritual of invoking and envisioning the deities. The gods (*deva*) were considered great allies from the invisible realm without whose benediction life could not run smoothly.

Yoga, in this sense, may already have been practiced in the native Indus civilization, which is said to predate the invasion of the Sanskrit-speaking Vedic tribes by a millennium.

Originally Hindu Yoga was tied to a polytheistic worldview. The Sanskrit word was generally interpreted in the sense of "yoking," from the verbal root *yuj* ("to yoke, harness"). What had to be yoked was attention, flitting from object to object. Only by focusing attention, by turning it into a laser beam, could the barrier between the visible and the invisible be crossed and the gods contacted.

Before long, however, Yoga's growing technology of physical and mental practices came to be associated with a nondualist (*advaita*) metaphysics. According to the earliest teachings of Hindu nondualism, as contained in the *Upanishads*, the multifaceted world is an emanation from the singular transcendental Reality called *brahman* ("that which thrives").[3] Yoga was introduced as a way back to that Singularity (*eka*).

That unitary Reality, which is supraconscious and utterly blissful, was experienced as the core not only of the whole universe but also of the human personality. As the core of the personality it was called "Self," or *atman*. The Sanskrit term *yoga* was accordingly redefined as the "union" between the lower or embodied self and the transcendental Self (*atman*), and this is still the prevalent understanding of the word inside and outside India. However, even Yoga as union includes an element of yoking, for we cannot realize the higher Self without proper focusing of attention.

With the exception of a single but influential school—that of

Classical Yoga—all Hindu schools of Yoga are based on the meta-physical idea of nonduality.[4] Classical Yoga, also called "Royal Yoga" (*raja-yoga*), was formulated by Patanjali some time in the second century A.D. As is obvious from his *Yoga-Sutra,* a work consisting of 195 short aphorisms (*sutra*), Patanjali taught a dualistic metaphysics. He pitted the Spirit or Self (in this school termed *purusha*) against Nature (*prakriti*). He regarded both as irreducible ultimate principles.

There are apparently many transcendental Selves, just as Nature comprises countless individual forms. However, only the Selves are conscious. Nature is insentient, and this includes the mind! The apparent consciousness of the mind (*citta*) is thought to be entirely due to the "proximity" of the Self's supraconscious awareness (*cit*). Nature and its products can never evolve to become the Self, and the Self does not emanate the different categories of Nature. Creation is a process whereby the transcendental foundation (*pradhana*) of Nature gives rise to lower levels and forms of existence.

The Self is merely a witness of this cosmic process, which runs its course automatically, just as the ultimate destruction of the visible and invisible universe is preprogrammed. The Self is neither born nor dies. It is indestructible because it does not consist of any parts. Only from the viewpoint of the unenlightened mind does the Self, or consciousness, appear to be implicated in Nature's realm.

For Patanjali, the purpose of Yoga was to extricate the Spirit from its apparent involvement in the processes of Nature. That involvement is a case of mistaken identity: The Self falsely identifies with the body-mind, thus causing the phenomenon of individuated consciousness, which suffers its presumed limitations.

Patanjali's dualist philosophy is unconvincing but it does have a certain practical merit because, from our finite viewpoint, the conscious subject, or Self, does indeed appear to be an "other" that must be carefully distinguished from the objective world and matter.

Through progressive discrimination (*viveka*), we cease to identify with what we in truth are not. Finally, the Self awakens to its true status as an eternally free and independent Consciousness. This condition is not merely an altered state of consciousness, because even high ecstatic states still occur within the orbit of Nature. Rather, Self-realization is an utterly transcendental "non-event." It is a non-event because the Self is never actually in bondage to Nature but is essentially and perpetually free. It only deems itself attached to a body-mind and therefore seemingly suffers all the limitations of embodiment. The whole drama of bondage followed by liberation is enacted on the stage of the mind alone.

In Classical Yoga, Self-realization is called *kaivalya*, which means literally "aloneness." That which is "alone" (*kevala*), or separate from Nature, is the transcendental Self. But the Self is not a windowless monad, which would be a dreary prospect and hardly worthy of the kind of sustained spiritual aspiration that marks all authentic Yoga. Although Patanjali says nothing about this, we must assume that the many eternal Selves are all copresent and thus intersecting in infinity. In Patanjali's understanding, Self-realization presupposes the demise of the body-mind. This is the ideal of *videha-mukti* or "disembodied liberation." Not surprisingly, one of the traditional commentators on his *Yoga-Sutra* defined Yoga as *viyoga* or "disunion," that is, separation.

By contrast, most nondualist schools of Yoga teach the ideal of *jivan-mukti* or "living liberation." According to this teaching, we do not need to die first before we can realize our true identity, the Self. Rather, liberation is a matter of recovering the Self in the midst of the hustle and bustle of life and then transforming life in the light of that realization. This is the ideal celebrated in the nondualist tradition of Vedanta, which has long been closely associated with Yoga.

Yoga, whether dualist or nondualist, is concerned with the elimination of suffering (*duhkha*). Here suffering does not mean the pain resulting from a cut or the emotional torment experienced through political oppression. These are simply manifestations of a deeper existential suffering. That suffering is the direct outcome of our habitual sense of being locked into a body-mind that is separate from all others. Yoga seeks to prevent future suffering of this kind by pointing the way to the unitary consciousness that is disclosed in ego-transcending ecstatic states.

From the viewpoint of traditional Yoga, even the pleasure or well-being (*sukha*) experienced as a result of the regular performance of yogic postures, breath control, or meditation is suffused with suffering. First of all, the pleasure is bound to be only temporary, whereas the innate bliss (*ananda*) of the Self is permanent.

Second, pleasure is relative: We can compare our present sense of enjoyment with similar experiences at different times or by different people. Thus, our experience contains an element of envy. Third, there is always the hidden fear that a pleasurable state will come to an end, which is a reasonable assumption.

Yoga is a systematic attempt to step out of this whole cycle of gain and loss. When the *yogin* or *yogini* is in touch with the Reality beyond the body-mind, and when he or she has a taste of the unalloyed delight of the Self, all possible pleasures that derive from objects (rather than the Self) come to lose their fascination. The mind begins to be more equanimous. As the *Bhagavad-Gita* (II.48), perhaps the greatest Yoga scripture, puts it: "Yoga is balance (*samatva*)."

This notion of balance is intrinsic to Yoga and occurs on many levels of the yogic work. Its culmination is in the "vision of sameness" (*sama-darshana*), which is the graceful state in which we see everything in the same light. Everything stands revealed as the great Reality, and nothing excites us as being more valuable than anything else. We regard a piece of gold and a clump of clay or a beautiful person and an unattractive individual with the same even-temperedness. Nor are we puffed up by praise or deflated by blame.

This condition, which is one of utter lucidity and serenity, must not be confused with one of the many types of ecstasy (*samadhi*) known to *yogins*. Ecstasies, visions, and psychic phenomena are not at all the point of spiritual life. They can and do occur when we earnestly devote ourselves to higher values, but they are by-products rather than the goal of authentic spirituality. They should certainly not be made the focus of our aspiration.

Thus, Yoga is a comprehensive *way of life* in which the transcendental Reality, or Divine, is given precedence over other concerns. It is a sacred path that conducts us, in the words of an ancient *Upanishad*, from the unreal to the Real, from falsehood to Truth, from the temporal to the Eternal.

The yogic way of life exists in two fundamental forms. One can be said to be marked by the mystical ascent from the ordinary consciousness to the supraconsciousness, as it is revealed at the peak of ecstasy, the state of *nirvikalpa-samadhi*. The Sanskrit word *nirvikalpa* can mean either "formless" or "beyond conception."

When the movements of the mind are completely pacified in the ecstatic state, the transcendental Reality flashes forth. The bliss of this temporary realization is so powerful and attractive that the *yogin* becomes quite indifferent to ordinary life and desires to spend more and more time in the state of transconceptual ecstasy (*nirvikalpa-samadhi*). This approach coincides with the way of external renunciation (*samnyasa*), consisting in the abandonment of the world. The second fundamental form of the yogic path does not lead away from the world in some mystical flight. On the contrary, it affirms life and creativity but brings a new perspective to them. This supramystical orientation is not primarily interested in the fleeting eclipse of the ego that mystical experience provides. It recognizes all experiences, including the elevated state of *nirvikalpa-samadhi*, as being merely that: an experience. Rather, it is based on the continuous transcendence of the ego to the point where the deliberate act of self-transcendence becomes a spontaneous gesture, which is known as *sahaja-samadhi*.

Because this second, supramystical form of the yogic path does not deny life, it also does not reject the faculty of reason, as is typically the case with mystical Yoga. This has been clearly understood and elaborated by the Western sage Paul Brunton, who drank deeply from the fountain of Hindu Yoga and Vedanta. In his *Notebooks* he wrote:

> It is not enough to negate thinking; this may yield a mental blank without content. We have also to transcend it. The first is the way of ordinary yoga; the second is the way of philosophic yoga. In the second way, therefore, we seek strenuously to carry thought to its most abstract and rarefied point, to a critical culminating whereby its whole character changes and it merges of its own accord in the higher source whence it arises. If successful, this produces a pleasant, sometimes ecstatic state—but the ecstasy is not our aim as with ordinary mysticism. With us the reflection must keep loyally to a loftier aim, that of dissolving the ego in its divine source.[5]

We certainly cannot *think* our way to spiritual liberation. The reflection Brunton speaks of is a matter of wisdom or higher understanding, called *jnana* in Sanskrit. This faculty corresponds to the Greek concept of *gnosis*, which is central to the esoteric tradition of

Gnosticism. Such higher understanding alone can guide us to a realization that is full and that, in turn, can transfigure our ordinary life. Then, whether we are visited by ecstasies or, as is inevitable, by experiences of sorrow and pain, we remain steadfast in our adherence to the all-encompassing Reality. Thus we succeed in bringing some of its glory and brilliance down to earth.

NOTES

1. The word *yogi*, which is often found in the English literature, represents the nominative case of the Sanskrit stem *yogin*. For the sake of consistency and easy recognition I have used the stem of Sanskrit words throughout this book. There are many different nominative case endings, which can be confusing to those not familiar with the Sanskrit language. For instance, the word *asana* ("seat" or "posture") becomes *asanam* in the nominative; *yoga* ("union") becomes *yogah*; go ("cow") becomes *gauh*; etc.

2. See G. Feuerstein, *Yoga: The Technology of Ecstasy* (Los Angeles: J.P. Tarcher, 1989).

3. For an explanation of the *Upanishads*, see the next essay.

4. Classical Yoga is explained in essays 8–10.

5. P. Brunton, *The Notebooks of Paul Brunton*. Vol. 1: *Perspectives: The Timeless Way of Wisdom* (Burdett, NY: Larson Publications, 1984), p. 261.

2

"THAT ART THOU"—
THE ESSENCE OF NONDUALIST VEDANTA

Gargi Vacaknavi approached the venerable Sage Yajnavalkya, asking him to instruct her.

"Ask, Gargi," he said.

"Across what is that which is above the sky and beneath the earth woven?" she asked.

"It is woven across space," replied Yajnavalkya.

"Across what, then, is space woven?" asked Gargi.

"That the initiates call the Imperishable. It is neither coarse nor fine, neither long nor short. Indeed, It is without measure. It casts no shadow, and there is no darkness in It. It is beyond space and energy. It is odorless, tasteless, and voiceless, as well as fearless, unaging, undying, and immortal. That Imperishable is the unseen Seer, the unheard Hearer, the unthought Thinker, the ununderstood Understander. Other than That there is nothing that sees, hears, thinks, or understands," replied Yajnavalkya.

This striking passage—here only paraphrased—is found in the ancient *Brihad-Aranyaka-Upanishad* (chapter III) dating back to perhaps 800 B.C. This is the oldest scripture of the Upanishadic genre. The *Upanishads* are Sanskrit works containing esoteric teachings about the "secret" of the transcendental Self, most of which were transmitted by word of mouth for countless generations until they were committed to writing in the Middle Ages.

Sage Yajnavalkya was an enlightened adept who taught the sublime wisdom of nonduality (*advaita*). We know very little about this illustrious sage, but the scant information we have about him suggests that he was one of ancient India's most remarkable spiritual teachers.

The esoteric teaching of nondualism can be summarized as follows. The manifold universe is, in truth, a Single Reality. There is only one Great Being, which the sages call *brahman*, in which all the countless forms of existence reside. That Great Being is utter Consciousness, and It is the very Essence, or Self (*atman*), of all beings. *Tat tvam asi*, "That art thou," is one of the great dicta of the *Upanishads*. It expresses the quintessence of their esotericism.

It is no accident that in this Sanskrit utterance the word *tat* ("that") precedes *tvam* ("thou"). Stylistic elegance is by no means the only explanation. As hinted at by Paul Brunton, there is a deeper significance as well.[1] And that significance is that the *tat* ontologically precedes the *tvam*. In other words, our individual life arises against the backdrop of the universal Reality and is in fact entirely dependent on it.

Since the One Being is our essential core, we can realize it, and it is realizable through proper discrimination (*viveka*) and renunciation (*vairagya*). By means of the former, we can hold apart that which is real from that which is unreal or illusory (that is, anything that is experienced as manifold rather than Single). By means of the latter, we can inwardly cleave to that which is Single (*eka*) and thereby recover our identity with it.

This, in a nutshell, is the position of Advaita Vedanta, which has for millennia been the most influential of all schools of Hinduism. In the West, its philosophical elegance and mystical cogency have attracted many distinguished thinkers—Schopenhauer, who regarded the study of the *Upanishads* as the solace of his life, Ralph Waldo Emerson, Walt Whitman, Gerald Heard, Aldous Huxley, and Julius Robert Oppenheimer.

Advaita Vedanta means "nondual Vedanta." Vedanta is literally "the end of the Vedas." This can be understood in at least two senses. First, Vedanta is, historically speaking, the tail end of the ancient revelation as embodied in the hymns of the four *Vedas*. Second, it is the final fulfillment of the Vedic revelation.

The *Vedas* are to Hinduism what the Old Testament is to Christianity. The Sanskrit word *veda* stands for knowledge, more precisely the sacred knowledge that is concerned with the archaic sacrificial ritual and the complex symbolism and mythology surrounding it.

With the *Upanishads*, just as with the New Testament in the

Middle East, a new spirit emerged in India. The knowledge that the sages of the *Upanishads* were communicating was gnostic or mystical in nature. They taught that the real sacrifice occurs on the level of the human psyche, or the human heart. And so they spoke of ways in which our everyday consciousness could be transformed and transcended, so that we would reawaken to our true identity—*as* the Self or *atman*.

The *Upanishads*, like the *Vedas*, are considered "revelation" or *shruti*. They are treasured as the words of inspired and enlightened adepts. Nondualism is the philosophy that is expressed in the *Upanishads*, the "Himalayas of the soul." There are now more than two hundred of these texts, and they continue to be composed by Hindu mystics to this day.

Many of the early *Upanishads* are in dialogue form, which gives us a sense of participating in the disclosure of the Upanishadic secrets. We encounter such charismatic wisdom teachers as Yajnavalkya, King Ajatashatru, and Uddalaka, who were once surely inaccessible to all but the most serious seekers after wisdom. It is quite amazing that today we can obtain inexpensive paperbacks that reveal what was once the most concealed esoteric teaching, whose price was certainly much higher than a few dollars: It called for obedience and submission to a teacher, often for many long, trying years, before anything at all was disclosed to the student. Perhaps because we think we can come by this wisdom so easily and cheaply, we generally don't *really* value it. For instance, how many of us have *actually* changed our lives after delving into these esoteric scriptures?

The transmission of the Upanishadic teachings was not merely a matter of passing on theories. Rather it involved the transmission of the spiritual force or presence of the teacher, who had at least glimpsed the Self, if not fully realized it. Hence the qualified aspirant was expected to be like an empty vessel into which the *guru*'s grace and wisdom could be poured. The Upanishadic sages showed little concern about justifying any of their teachings philosophically, precisely because their verity could be demonstrated to the initiate through direct transmission.

Only as other metaphysical traditions—both Hindu and non-Hindu—started to rival Advaita Vedanta, did the Vedanta teachers have to become more sophisticated philosophers and defenders of their faith. At this point, Vedanta became one of the six "systems" or *darshanas* (lit., "viewpoints") of Hinduism. The six orthodox Hindu viewpoints are Samkhya, Yoga, Vaisheshika, Nyaya, Mimamsa, and Vedanta.

Samkhya (the name means "number") is often considered the oldest of the Hindu traditions. It consists essentially in an effort to describe the major patterns of existence. The Samkhya teachers developed an evolutionary theory and introduced the distinction between the principle of Consciousness or Spirit (*purusha*) and the principle of insentient Nature (*prakriti*), arguing that whereas the former is immutable, the latter is constantly changing.

Yoga, which largely adopted the Samkhya view of the world, was primarily a practical path of discovering, or recovering, transcendental Consciousness by means of moral, bodily, and mental disciplines.

Vedanta taught, as we have seen, the essential Oneness of everything. The three viewpoints—Samkhya, Yoga, and Vedanta—were originally closely allied and became separate traditions only in the course of many centuries.

The Vaisheshika school of thought was a kind of naturalist philosophy that, like Samkhya, tried to make sense of the phenomenal world.

The Nyaya viewpoint was essentially a system of logic, closely associated with the Vaisheshika.

Finally, the Mimamsa school of thought was a form of ritualist philosophy that sought to justify the Vedic sacrificial cult. It is also known as the "Earlier Vedanta" or Purva Vedanta, whereas the teachings of the Upanishadic sages came to be known as "Later Vedanta" or Uttara Vedanta.

These six "systems," which have their own schools and subschools, make up the orthodox fold of Hindu philosophy. Then there are also unorthodox schools of Hinduism—like materialism—that are so classified because they deny the Vedic revelation outright.

Facing these different branches of Hinduism were such ramifying traditions as Jainism and Buddhism. Gautama, the founder of Buddhism, appears to have studied under Samkhya and Yoga teachers. He rejected idealistic metaphysics, of the Vedantic type, and instead preached a kind of pragmatic realism. Yet, later Buddhist teachers, especially Asanga and Vasubandhu, elaborated idealistic schools of thought that closely resemble Advaita Vedanta. At any rate, all these different teachings cross-fertilized one another. For instance, Gaudapada—Shankara's teacher's teacher—has often been called a hidden (Mahayana-) Buddhist, as has Shankara himself.

The earliest extant (though not the earliest known) systematic treatment of Vedanta is Badarayana's *Vedanta-Sutra*, which is also known as *Brahma-Sutra*. This compilation, dating back to around 200 A.D., was an attempt to reconcile the various Vedanta traditions. Primarily it was based on the principal *Upanishads* and the *Bhagavad-Gita*, which, as few people realize, is traditionally considered an *Upanishad*.

The *Upanishads*, the *Gita*, and the *Vedanta-Sutra* are the scriptural foundation of all later Vedanta schools. Any teacher wishing to establish his own school would write commentaries on all of them. This is exactly what Shankara (788–820 A.D.), the greatest proponent of Advaita Vedanta, did. His school is known as Kevala Advaita or Absolute Nondualism, because of its extreme position relative to the illusory nature of the perceived world. Today when Vedanta is mentioned, generally Shankara's school is intended. This is not altogether fair, since other schools—particularly Ramanuja's Vishishta Advaita or Qualified Nondualism—have large followings as well. But Shankara's philosophical system has been found so attractive because it is deemed the most self-consistent.

Yet, although Shankara was clearly a remarkable man, his genius lay perhaps not so much in the field of philosophy as in the areas of theology and practical spirituality. Much of what tends to be attributed to him was actually established by his teachers, though he brought to it an astounding breadth and depth of learning. But Shankara was, first and foremost, an accomplished *yogin* and Self-realizer, who commanded the respect and veneration of his monastic and lay followers, as well as the intelligentsia of his day.

Whereas his Sanskrit commentaries on the *Upanishads*, the *Brahma-Sutra*, and the *Bhagavad-Gita* tend to be as dry as many Christian scholastic treatises, his more popular works reflect his great wisdom and practical experience as a meditator and an ecstatic. His *Upadesha-Sahasri* ("Thousand Instructions") and *Viveka-*

Cudamani ("Crest Jewel of Discrimination") can be especially recommended.

It is Shankara's Absolute Nondualism that, in our century, had its most charismatic representative in the person of the South Indian sage Ramana Maharshi (1879–1950). He was introduced to Western seekers mainly through the works of Paul Brunton and Arthur Osborne. Sri Ramana spontaneously awakened at the age of sixteen and for the rest of his life remained stably in *sahaja-samadhi*, or natural ecstasy.

In recent years, the Marathi sage Nisargadatta Maharaj (1897–1981) has demonstrated to us that Advaita Vedanta is not merely hearsay or an antiquated philosophy, but a living tradition of God-realization. Unlike Ramana Maharshi, who was a life-long ascetic, Sri Nisargadatta lived as a householder, quietly going about his daily business, all the while attracting a growing number of seekers.

Like Sri Ramana, Nisargadatta asked his students to deeply enquire of themselves: "Who am I?" In Socratic fashion, he guided them to the point where, if they were at all open, they could intuit—however briefly and incompletely—the great Mystery that there is only "I" and no "me" or "other." That "I" is, of course, not the ego-sense but the transcendental "I-am-ness," the I AM, the Self-Identity, which Ramana Maharshi also called "I-ness" and *aham-vritti.*

The similarity between their teachings is not accidental either. For if there is indeed only the One Reality that we, in our unenlightenment, habitually fragment into subject and object, then we can talk about it rationally only in a limited number of ways. But, perhaps, by talking about it, as we are fond of doing, we only distract ourselves from the real business at hand: to realize that single Identity in every moment and with every breath. Therefore both teachers agree that, in the end, silence is the best policy. It obliges us to simply be present as That.

NOTE

1. See P. Brunton, *The Notebooks of Paul Brunton.* Vol. 10: *The Orient: Its Legacy to the West* (Burdett, NY: Larson Publications, 1987.)

3

EAST COMES WEST: A HISTORICAL PERSPECTIVE

"Since the Renaissance there has been no event of such world-wide significance in the history of culture as the discovery of Sanskrit literature in the latter part of the eighteenth century."[1] This pronouncement was made in the year 1900 by the renowned British Sanskritist Arthur A. Macdonell, who wrote the first comprehensive history of Sanskrit literature in English. Events since then have amply borne out the professor's reading of the situation.

Yoga and Vedanta have been a part of the kaleidoscope of Western culture for nearly a hundred years. Britain was the first European country to open its doors to India's spiritual heritage and bid welcome to the new twentieth-century breed of proselytizing Hindus. After centuries, if not millennia, of almost perfect self-chosen centripetal existence, India's spiritual paragons finally resolved to break their long silence and spread the gospel outside their homeland.

The early involvement of the British people with Yoga and Vedanta is not completely surprising considering Britain's long-standing contact with India, beginning with the establishment of the East India Company on the last day of the year 1600. It was Warren Hastings, the founder of the British *raj* in India, who inadvertently initiated Indic studies and the various other novel academic disciplines arising as a result of this scholarly preoccupation with Indic society and culture.

Realizing the advantages of a policy that would respect the native social and religious customs and mores as far as possible, Hastings ordered the compilation of a comprehensive treatise on indigenous law in Sanskrit. Since the sacred language of the brahmins (*brahmana*), the custodians of Hinduism, was at that time still a jealously guarded secret, this work had first to be translated into Persian before it could be rendered into English in 1776. There simply were no linguists who were competent enough in Sanskrit to measure up to the task at hand.

The very first Englishman to acquire a thorough knowledge of Sanskrit, at the instigation of Hastings, was Charles Wilkins. Previously only a handful of Christian missionaries had, for obvious reasons, made an attempt to learn this sophisticated language of the educated Hindus. As early as 1785, Wilkins published his translation of the *Bhagavad-Gita* ("Lord's Song"), the most celebrated of all Hindu scriptures and at the same time an acclaimed Yoga classic. It was the first of a large number of other renderings of this beautiful Sanskrit tract. According to the Gita Press in Gorakhpur (Northern India), there exist more than one thousand editions of the *Gita*, and it has been translated into more than thirty languages.

Another early pioneer of Sanskrit Studies was William Jones (1746–1794), founder of the Asiatic Society of Bengal, who brought out several important translations of legal and literary texts in Sanskrit, as well as a rendering of the enchanting *Isha-Upanishad* ("Secret Teaching of the Lord"), published posthumously in 1799. The *Isha-Upanishad* is a succinct poetic statement of the principles of Vedanta metaphysics.

A scholar with encyclopedic knowledge was Henry Thomas Colebrooke (1765–1837), who, among other things, published in 1837 the very first treatment of Yoga by a Westerner.

Serendipity was responsible for bringing Sanskrit studies to Germany. While traveling through France, the Englishman Alexander Hamilton (1765–1824) fell victim to Napoleon's hostile policy against the British. Kept prisoner in Paris, he taught Sanskrit to other scholars, including Friedrich Schlegel, the German romantic poet who then co-founded with Franz Bopp the discipline of comparative philology. Schlegel enthusiastically maintained that the pinnacle of Romanticism was to be found in India, the "source of all languages, all the thoughts and poems of the human spirit." [2]

The virgin science of Indic studies (Indology) made a tremendous impact on the thinking of Hegel, Schopenhauer, and Nietzsche. A conveniently tailored knowledge of India's heritage was also an important contributary to Nazi ideology, with its myth of Aryan supremacy—a telling example of how even the most excellent knowledge can be put to destructive use.[3]

For a long time academic philosophy ignored India's intellectual contribution. This has changed somewhat in our own century. Encyclopedias and dictionaries of philosophy now generally include entries on Indic thought. Perhaps philosophers like J. Royce, G. Santayana, and W.E. Hocking, who were appreciative of India's philosophical legacy, have had some influence in this. But the real interest in India lies in the popular sector, as we will shortly see.

To get back to Schlegel. His romantic enthusiasm was fully shared, among others, by F. Max Müller (1823–1900), one of the great German scholars, who lived and taught in England for most of his life. Apart from being an accomplished Sanskrit scholar, Müller was also founder of the discipline of comparative mythology. Though he remained faithful to a liberally understood Christianity, Müller considered the nondualist philosophy of Vedanta as "a system in which human speculation seems . . . to have reached its very acme." [4] Müller also remarked:

> Before we begin to scoff at the Yoga and its minute treatment of postures, breathings, and other means of mental concentration, we ought first of all to try to understand their original intention. Everything can become absurd by exaggeration, and this has been, no doubt, the case with the self-imposed discipline and tortures of the Yogins [read: fakirs]. But originally their object seems to have been no other than to counteract the distractions of the senses. We all consider the closing of the eyelids and the stopping of the ears against disturbing noises useful for serious meditation. This was the simple beginning of Yoga . . . If we ourselves must admit that our senses and all that they imply are real obstacles to quiet meditation, the attempts to reduce these sensuous affections to some kind of quietude or equability (Samatva) need not surprise us, nor need we be altogether incredulous as to the marvellous results obtained by means of ascetic exercises by Yogins in India, as little as we should treat the visions of St. Francis or St. Teresa as downright impositions. The real relation of the soul to the body and of the senses to the soul is still as great a mystery to us as it was to the ancient Yogins of India, and their experiences, if only honestly related, deserve certainly the same careful attention as the stigmata of Roman Catholic saints. They may be or they may not be true, but there is no reason why they should be treated as *a priori* untrue. From this point of view it seems to me that the Yoga-philosophy deserves some attention on the part of philosophers, more particularly of the physical school of psychologists . . .[5]

India was and still is impressed with Müller's great empathy for India's spiritual heritage. Even today Hindu traditionalists venerate him as something of a saint. Several eminent Hindu authorities pilgrimaged to his home in England.

The first of them was Keshub Chandra Sen, the third leader of the Brahmo Samaj reform movement founded by Rammohan Roy in 1828. Sen arrived in Britain in 1870, and his campaign did much to further augment the dialogue between India and the West.

But it was Rammohan Roy who not only pioneered what is known as the modern Hindu "renaissance" but who was the very first modern Hindu to embark on the forbidden journey across the ocean. He came to England in 1831, and died there two years later. Roy translated the *Vedanta-Sara* ("Essence of Nondualism") and several *Upanishads* first into his native Bengali and then into English. He made an immense impression on the educated sections of British society, and also greatly inspired the American Transcendentalists, notably Ralph Waldo Emerson.

Then followed the spectacular visit of Swami Vivekananda (1863–1902) to America in 1893. He was the favorite and most famous disciple of the Hindu visionary Ramakrishna, who was celebrated in Bengal as an "incarnation" (*avatara*) of the Divine. For Vivekananda, his *guru* Ramakrishna embodied all that is best in the age-old tradition of Hinduism. He went further than that, claiming that Ramakrishna's presence in the world signaled the beginning of another golden age. Vivekananda thus became the first representative of Neo-Hinduism.

Largely through Vivekananda's efforts, the encounter between India and the West became a practical rather than a theoretical affair. He had a fine mind but was not a scholar limited by any academic ambitions. He did not want merely to interpret India's wisdom to the West but rather to change people's hearts and usher them into a spiritual way of life.

Vivekananda went to Chicago to speak at the World Parliament of Religions in Chicago. He had not been invited, nor did he have any friends when he first arrived in the United States but relied solely on his sense of destiny. Through a series of fortunate "coincidences," he, a thirty-year-old unknown Hindu, was elected to address the assembly on behalf of his entire culture.

Vivekananda   *Ramakrishna*

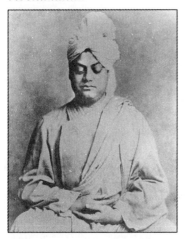
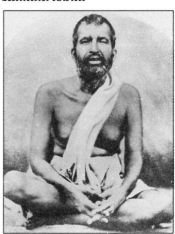

Vivekananda's frank and heartfelt manner and the clarity of his exposition of the principles of Hinduism greatly impressed his American audience. The *New York Herald* styled him as "undoubtedly the greatest figure in the Parliament of Religions." He delivered ten or twelve stirring speeches, which left many people galvanized and awed. Subsequently Vivekananda went on lecture tours around the country, establishing small pockets of spiritually motivated individuals. His writings were still more influential, reaching the minds and hearts of great men like William James and Leo Tolstoy.

In the summer of 1896, Vivekananda met Max Müller in England. This was his second visit to the British Isles. He thought highly of Müller, and the Sanskritist reciprocated those warm feelings. Two years later, Müller published his book *Ramakrishna: His Life and Sayings*, which was based on the recollections of Vivekananda and other disciples of Ramakrishna. In his preface, Müller, forever championing India's cause, wrote:

> From such sayings we learn that though the real presence of the Divine in nature and in the human soul was nowhere felt so strongly and so universally as in India, and though the fervent love of God, nay the sense of complete absorption in the Godhead, has nowhere found a stronger and more eloquent expression than in the utterances of Ramakrishna, yet he perfectly knew the barriers that separate divine and human nature.
>
> If we remember that these utterances of Ramakrishna reveal to

us not only his own thoughts, but the faith and hope of millions of human beings, we may indeed feel hopeful about the future of that country. The consciousness of the Divine in man is there, and is shared by all, even by those who seem to worship idols. This constant sense of the presence of God is indeed the common ground on which we may hope that in time not too distant the great temple of the future will be erected, in which Hindus and non-Hindus may join hands and hearts in worshipping the same Supreme Spirit— who is not far from every one of us, for in Him we live and move and have our being.[6]

Swami Vivekananda's instant success seems to have fulfilled his guru's prophecy that he would shake the foundations of the world. Certainly without his missionary work, the counterculture of the 1960s and 1970s would have been different, for Vedanta and Yoga were prominent features of the countercultural quake.

Three years after Swami Vivekananda's address to the Parliament of Religions, another Hindu pilgrim made his way across the ocean. He was Govindananda Bharati, who arrived in England in 1896 and stayed there for five years. During his residence he was granted no fewer than eighteen audiences by Queen Victoria.

In 1902, another much-loved sage, Swami Rama Tirtha (1873– 1906), went to America where he stayed for two years and became quite influential. He was an orphaned child who, by his single-mindedness and native brilliance, became a professor of mathematics of rare distinction. At the end of 1900, when in his late twenties, he renounced the world and started his mendicant life in the Himalayas.

Having discovered the still point within himself, Rama Tirtha felt moved to share his peace with his "brothers" and "sisters" outside India. He made his new home in California, where he founded a retreat center on Mount Shasta. His lectures were gathered in three volumes entitled *In Woods of God-Realisation*. Thus Rama Tirtha was among the first of a long stream of Hindus to preach abroad—a stream that continues to flow.

By the turn of the century, Yoga and Vedanta were no longer the unknown quantities that they had been to the early missionaries or even the founding fathers of Indology, who had little more than ridicule for it. Largely thanks to the publishing efforts of the Theosophical Society founded by Helena Petrovna Blavatsky in 1875, students of India's wisdom now had reasonably accurate translations of a number of the more important Yoga scriptures.

These translations included the *Bhagavad-Gita*, the *Yoga-Vasishtha*, the *Yoga-Sutra*, several *Upanishads* dealing with Yoga, and the three principal scriptures of *hatha-yoga*, namely the *Hatha-Yoga-Pradipika*, the *Gheranda-Samhita*, and the *Shiva-Samhita*. As a matter of fact, comparatively few renderings of Yoga works have appeared since then.

Western students of Yoga were even given access to the more esoteric teachings of *kundalini-yoga* and Tantrism through the writings of Sir John Woodroffe (1865–1936), who also published under the pseudonym Arthur Avalon. Woodroffe, a retired High-Court judge in India, almost single-handedly reversed the prevailing scholarly prejudice against Tantrism. His many ground-breaking works, notably his translation of the *Mahanirvana-Tantra* (published in 1913 under the title *Tantra of the Great Liberation*), *Shakti and Shakta* (1918), and *The Serpent Power* (1919), brought to light teachings that, out of ignorance, were repudiated and denied by native Hindus but that belong to the most daring and noteworthy efforts of India's spiritual genius.

In the 1920s, the first popular expositions of Yoga saw the light of day in English and in German. The numerous works of "Ramacharaka" were widely read. This Sanskrit name belonged to a former lawyer, William Warren Atkinson (1862–1932), who had left his stressful law practice in Chicago to study Yoga in India and returned to the States to spread the good news. There were other professionals who likewise pilgrimaged to the East for illumination. Among them was Theos Bernard, who studied with Yogendra Mastanami in Bombay. Bernard's experiment with *hatha-yoga* is faithfully described in his 1947 book *Hatha-Yoga: The Report of a Personal Experience*, which served as an important sourcebook in the 1950s and 1960s.

Bernard's teacher, Yogendra, was a disciple of the long-lived Paramahamsa Madhavadasa (1798–1921). Yogendra visited America in 1919, and greatly inspired Benedict Lust, the founder of naturopathy. He also instructed Pierre Bernard, Theos Bernard's uncle, who was possibly the first Tantric in America.

Another well-known disciple of Madhavadasa was Swami

Kuvalayananda (1883–1966), who founded the Kaivalyadhama Ashram and Research Institute in 1921. Kuvalayananda, who pioneered physical education in India, was a tireless researcher. He believed that Yoga should and could be studied scientifically. The numerous experiments conducted by him and his research team clearly demonstrated that *yogins* were capable of an astonishing control over their bodily functions, including some of the processes of the autonomic nervous system.

Kuvalayananda's scientific endeavors were made more widely known through the book *Yoga: A Scientific Evaluation,* authored by Kovoor T. Behanan and first published in 1937. Behanan summarized his investigation with these words:

> Whatever may be one's opinion of the yogic theory of the mind and its evolution, its success in developing a healthy emotional equilibrium is empirically verifiable. Nor does one need to reach the higher stages of its practices to attain this desirable adjustment . . . As far as the metaphysical tenets of yoga are concerned, they are an audacious and poetic leap in the dark—worthy enough to occupy a spacious hall in the "Mansions of Philosophy" that the human mind has spun in its irresistible desire to explain the warp and woof of the unknown. [7]

In the West, *hatha-yoga* was popularized as a system promising vigorous health, physical control, and prolonged youth. In England, after World War II, it was above all the television broadcasts by Sir Paul Dukes (1889–1967) that sustained and accelerated the public interest in Yoga. At that time Yoga was added to the curriculum of Further Education.

In 1950, Selvarajan Yesudian arrived in Switzerland to teach physical Yoga. His book *Sport und Yoga* was translated into fourteen languages with more than 500,000 copies sold.

Also in the middle of our century, *hatha-yoga* was popularized in America by the Russian-born Eugenie Petersen, who is better known as Indra Devi. She is sometimes called the "First Lady of Yoga in America." She had fallen ill with an allegedly incurable heart disease but managed to cure herself in one week through yogic healing, and this astonishing success prompted her to study Yoga and subsequently teach it in Shanghai, India, and America.

Indra Devi studied under Sri Tirumalai Krishnamacharya (1891–1989), a Sanskrit scholar and naturopath and personal Yoga instructor

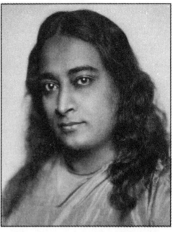

Yogananda

of the Maharaja of Mysore. Krishnamacharya traced his spiritual lineage back to the tenth-century South Indian adept Nathamuni, who practiced the eightfold Yoga and authored, among other scriptures, the *Yoga-Rahasya* ("Secret Doctrine of Yoga").

Krishnamacharya was also the *guru* of his son T.K.V. Desikachar and his brother-in-law B.K.S. Iyengar, who both have flourishing centers in various countries around the world. Iyengar (b. 1918) has trained more than five hundred teachers, and his system, which emphasizes flexibility and strength, is the most prominent force in American *hatha-yoga* today.

The amazing bodily control that can be achieved through *hatha-yoga* has been amply demonstrated by Swami Rama, who came to the United States in 1970. His yogic abilities were extensively tested at the Menninger Foundation. A popular account of that project, which was conducted by Elmer and Alyce Green, can be found in Doug Boyd's book *Swami.*[8]

Since the first quarter of the twentieth century countless Westerners have turned to *hatha-yoga*, but there were also those who steeped themselves in the art of meditation. Not a few were attracted to the charismatic personality of Paramahansa Yogananda (1893–1952) and found his *kriya-yoga* particularly helpful. This Yoga is said to be a form of *raja-yoga* ("Royal Yoga"), focusing on meditation.

Yogananda arrived in Boston, Massachusetts, in 1920 to address

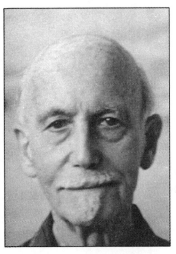

Paul Brunton

the International Congress of Religious Liberals. Like Vivekananda before him, he used the public interest created by his speech to tour the country fairly extensively. Five years later, he founded the Self-Realization Fellowship in Los Angeles, attracting tens of thousands of students at the time. Today the Fellowship claims a worldwide membership of more than a million followers.

The spiritual dimension of Yoga and Vedanta was also championed by Paul Brunton (1898–1981), a former journalist and editor, whose own spiritual transformation over the years is evident from his writings and photographs as well as the tranquil manner of his death. Brunton's eleven books have been widely read since the 1930s. It was his first work, *A Search In Secret India* (1934), which made the sage Sri Ramana Maharshi of Tiruvannamalai famous in the West. In recent years (1984–1988), Brunton's invaluable *Notebooks* were published in sixteen volumes.

We also must not forget the lofty spiritual philosophy of Sri Aurobindo (1872–1950), which made an impact especially in more intellectual circles. Prominent spokesmen for Aurobindo's spiritual teachings were philosopher Haridas Chaudhuri, orientalist Frederic Spiegelberg, and the famous Harvard sociologist Pitirim A. Sorokin. Aurobindo's Integral Yoga seeks to overcome the one-sidedness of the ascetical ideal of traditional Hinduism and to incorporate the ideal of creativity into the spiritual process. Together with Sarvepalli

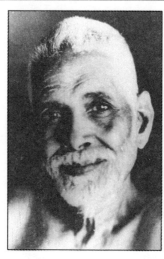

Ramana

Radhakrishnan (1888–1975), the former president of the Indian Republic, Aurobindo is regarded by many as modern India's finest philosopher. Both thinkers were keenly interested in dialoguing with the West, but neither adopted a missionizing stance. The same holds true of "Mahatma" M.K. Gandhi (1869–1948), whose adherence to the ideal of *karma-yoga,* the Yoga of self-transcending action, helped bring about India's independence one year before his assassination.

The Yoga-Vedanta movement reached its peak of popularity in the 1960s, which witnessed the emergence of the Beatles and Maharishi Mahesh Yogi, psychotomimetic drugs like LSD, and the incredible resurgence of occultism and paganism. Maharishi Mahesh Yogi's Transcendental Meditation (TM) became an overnight vogue, attracting large numbers of people. This is a form of *mantra-yoga,* which uses repetitive sound as a vehicle for concentration and relaxation. More than any other yogic teaching, Transcendental Meditation has provoked the greatest interest in the scientific community.

The modern Yoga and Vedanta movement in the West would be unthinkable without the swamis who were trained by Swami Shivananda (1887–1963) of Rishikesh. This former medical doctor renounced the world at the age of thirty-seven. He founded the Divine Life Society in 1939, which today has more than four hundred branches throughout the world. Among his students are Yogi Gupta, who arrived in America in 1954; the enterprising Vishnudevananda, who arrived in San Francisco four years later; Satyananda, a Tantric adept and founder of the Bihar School of Yoga, whose numerous disciples can be found in all parts of the world; the saintly Chidananda, whose best known American student is Lilias Folan, made famous by her PBS television series *Lilias, Yoga & You,* broadcast between 1970 and 1979; Satchidananda, one of the main holy figures of the Woodstock era; and the German-born woman Swami Sivananda Radha, founder of the Yasodhara Ashram in Canada.

Swami Muktananda (1908–1983) came to America in 1970, and during his lifetime established more than 350 Siddha Yoga Centers around the world. Equally popular was Bhagwan Shree Rajneesh (1931–1990), a former professor of philosophy, whose quasi-Tantric teachings appealed to tens of thousands of Westerners disgruntled with their sex-negative Christian heritage.

In the early 1980s, Rajneesh addressed daily some six thousand Westerners who had flocked to his retreat center in Poona, India, the "Esalen of the East." By 1985, when his empire began to crumble, he had a following of about twenty thousand Europeans and Americans. The scandals surrounding Rajneesh, however, were largely responsible for the widespread disillusionment with *guru*-centric Eastern traditions.

According to an informed guess there are today in Western countries several million Yoga and Vedanta enthusiasts. This phenomenon must be viewed together with the Western followings of other Eastern traditions, such as Buddhism, Zen, Taoism, and Sufism. Understandably, there is a certain anxiety among Christian clerics about these "imports." What they choose to forget, however, is that Christianity itself has its roots in the East. It started as a small sect within Judaism and then spread through the Roman Empire fairly rapidly.

According to one school of thought, Jesus of Nazareth went to India during the years about which the Bible remains silent. There he was initiated into the esoteric teachings of Hinduism. Apparently, in Kashmir there is a grave in which a certain Issa, who is identified by some as the adept Jesus, is supposed to lie.

Be that as it may, in its origin Jesus' teaching was as esoteric as Yoga and Vedanta once were. These metaphysical traditions were communicated by word of mouth and were accompanied by the gift of spiritual transmission, or what in the Christian tradition is known as spiritual baptism. Today few Christians have even an inkling about the esotericism of their own tradition. But this hidden dimension is a real meeting point between Christianity and Eastern traditions like Yoga and Vedanta.

Hence more mystically oriented Christians, like Father Bede Griffith or the monastic J.-M. Dechanet see no difficulty in melting Hindu practice with Christian doctrine. The latter wrote:

> I have never had any intention of founding an "order of Christian yogis" (although I have thought of bringing together a kind of fraternity of people who wanted to practise Yoga in the spirit I have suggested). I *do* think, however, that Yoga offers what is needed to bring about a complete renewal in the Latin West. Surely the day is not far off when those who are willing to submit to its austere discipline will be recognized for their authentic Christian life, their evangelical meekness, their sense of justice: in short, for their integrity and their sincerity. [9]

Even among those who are sympathetic toward Eastern traditions, few share Dechanet's optimism about the compatibility of Yoga with Christianity. What is clear, though, is that the ecumenical dialogue between East and West remains relatively barren so long as it is carried out exclusively on the level of the intellect. Dechanet's practical approach, demanding a personal commitment to the underlying spiritual process, is obviously more fruitful and also more interesting. For all mystical teachings are the product of actual experiences, and personal practice is the real key to understanding them.

According to the well-known Latin aphorism *ex oriente lux*, the Orient is the source of light. The sun rises in the east, and the cultural East is also the source of the world religions. But today, with the emergence of a global human culture, the distinction between East and West in cultural terms is no longer as relevant as it once was. We know that religious life was pursued for tens of thousands of years in the West prior to the arrival of Christianity, just as spirituality has been an integral part of the oft-forgotten "South," epitomized by the huge continent of Africa.

More than ever, we are challenged to transcend geographical, national, and racial boundaries and to discover the light within our own being—a light that is not determined by the compass needle but is omnipresent. Yoga and Vedanta, like Christianity, are simply paths to that universal light. They will trigger a resonance in some people but not in others. Only mutual understanding, respect, and tolerance can prevent us from veiling that light in each other.

NOTES

1. A.A. Macdonell, *A History of Sanskrit Literature* (London: William Heinemann, 1900), p. 1.

2. Cited from a letter dated September 15, 1803, in H. Ludeke, ed., *L. Tieck und die Brüder Schlegel* (Frankfurt, 130), p. 140.

3. The Sanskrit-speaking tribesmen who are said to have invaded the north of India about 1500 B.C. called themselves *arya* (meaning "noble").

4. M. Müller, *The Six Systems of Indian Philosophy* (London: Longman, Green and Co., 1916), p. v. First published in 1899, this book was Müller's last larger work, completed only two months before his death.

5. *Ibid.*, pp. 311–312.

6. F. Max Müller, *Ramakrishna: His Life and Sayings* (London: Longmans, Green, and Co., repr. 1916), pp. ix–x.

7. K.T. Behanan, *Yoga: A Scientific Evaluation* (New York: Dover Publications, repr. 1964), pp. 246–249.

8. See D. Boyd, *Swami* (New York: Paragon House, repr. 1990).

9. J.-M. Dechanet, *Yoga and God: An Invitation to Christian Yoga* (St. Meinrad, IN: Abbey Press, 1975), p. 161.

4

IN PRAISE OF STUDY

"Knowledge is power." But is it? I think this popular maxim is grossly misstated. Nevertheless, knowledge that leads to self-understanding is invaluable, because it is self-understanding that em-powers us in a certain sense: It empowers us to live a life that is not dictated by the mechanisms of our unconscious. And this is what Yoga, Vedanta, and all other spiritual traditions are ultimately concerned about.

Hence in the Yoga tradition, study is considered an important means to self-knowledge. It is known as *svadhyaya*. This Sanskrit word means literally "one's own going into"—from *sva* ("own"), *adhi* ("unto, into"), and *aya* "going." What it stands for is the serious and systematic study of the Yoga tradition. By confronting the tenets of Yoga, the student necessarily comes to inspect his or her own values and attitudes. Thus, *svadhyaya* is a yogic discipline, and is indeed listed as one of the five "restraints" (*niyama*). Such study is meant to be a journey of self-discovery, self-understanding, and self-transcendence.

In the Vedanta tradition, study is likewise deemed vitally important. It is called *shravana* or "hearing," which is the thoughtful reception of the sacred teachings. It leads to the conviction that there is indeed only the single Reality, without a trace of duality. This conviction is further strengthened through reflection (*manana*) and meditation (*nididhyasana*).

Yoga does not call for blind faith. Mere belief cannot help you realize that which abides beyond the conditional or egoic personality. It cannot enlighten you. Instead, Yoga has always been intensely experimental and experiential. And study is an integral part of this pragmatic orientation.

In the *Vishnu-Purana* (VI.6.2), an old encyclopedic Sanskrit work, we read: "From study one should proceed to practice (*yoga*) and from practice to study. The supreme Self is revealed through perfection in study *and* practice."

Many people, especially those with a dominant right brain, shy away from study. They would much rather learn a new breathing technique or polish their performance of one or another posture. Yet we have to apply and develop both hemispheres of our brain.

A purely left-brained approach to Yoga is therefore just as futile. "Armchair Yoga" can hardly replace actual experience. As the Yoga scriptures emphasize again and again, mere book knowledge is barren. In Yoga, theory and practice form a continuum, like space-time. Yoga is balance (*samatva*), as the *Bhagavad-Gita* (II.48) reminds us.

An ancient Hindu scripture, the *Shata-Patha-Brahmana* (XI.5.7.1), declares that for the serious student, study is a source of joy. It focuses the student's mind and lets him or her sleep peacefully. It also yields insight and the capacity to master life. What more could anyone ask for?

Especially for a Westerner following the Yoga tradition, it is important that he or she becomes steeped in the Yoga heritage. How else can you be sure that what you are doing is authentic Yoga? It will do us little good to use this or that meditation technique, or engage this or that physical practice, without knowing their deeper purposes and the philosophical presuppositions on which they are based.

Part of our study of Yoga must be to become thoroughly acquainted with the literature of this age-old tradition. The good news is that many of the Yoga texts, originally composed in Sanskrit, are available in English translations.

Ideally, you should read every single Yoga scripture available in English. Best begin at the beginning. Looking at the entire literature of Yoga, one can distinguish three broad historical categories: Pre-Classical (Upanishadic nondualist teachings), Classical (Patanjali's dualist school), and Post-Classical (nondualist traditions subsequent to Patanjali).

The scriptures of what can be called Pre-Classical Yoga precede the famous *Yoga-Sutra* of Patanjali, which was composed in the first centuries after Christ and which has come to be appreciated as the classical expression of the yogic tradition. These early texts teach a type of Vedanta Yoga according to which the ultimate Reality is a single continuum of blissful Being-Consciousness.

The oldest work in this category is the *Katha-Upanishad*, which belongs to the fourth or fifth century B.C. It contains the earliest reference to Yoga, outlining its basic practices and ideas. There are several reasonably reliable translations of this *Upanishad*, notably the readily available renderings by Sarvepalli Radhakrishnan and R.E. Hume. Since this text, like so many of the Yoga and Vedanta scriptures, is at times rather obscure, you may also want to consult Krishna Prem's insightful book *The Yoga of the Kathopanishad*.

While working through the *Katha-Upanishad*, it would profit you also to look at the *Shvetashvatara-Upanishad* and the *Maitrayaniya-Upanishad*, which are somewhat younger and so show the next stage in the evolution of Yoga. Again the translations of Radhakrishnan and Hume will serve you well.

The principal scripture of Pre-Classical Yoga is the widely read *Bhagavad-Gita*, which is the "New Testament" of Hinduism. Few people know that it is traditionally considered to be an *Upanishad*, that is, a secret doctrine that has been revealed rather than authored by a human individual. Technically, the *Gita* is an integral part of the *Mahabharata*, which is one of India's two great national epics— the other being the *Ramayana* of Valmiki.

Translations of the *Gita*, a wonderfully melodious Sanskrit work, abound. Some of the more popular ones, however, leave much to be desired. I can recommend the renderings by S. Radhakrishnan, R.C. Zaehner, and Krishna Prem (for his fine commentary written from a practitioner's point of view).

To really appreciate this work, you should definitely acquaint yourself with the broader cultural and historical background from which it emerged. Here I may refer you to my own introduction to the *Gita*, which is being used in college courses.

Pre-Classical materials are also contained in other sections of the *Mahabharata*, such as the *Moksha-Dharma* ("Liberation Doctrine") and the *Anugita* ("Secondary Song"). Unfortunately, these sections are not readily accessible, though students may search out F. Edgerton's *The Beginnings of Indian Philosophy*, which contains excerpts from the *Moksha-Dharma*. Of course, you can always tackle R.C. Roy's translation of the entire *Mahabharata*. Yogic materials are found especially in books VI, XII, and XIII of this mammoth work.

Next read and work through the *Yoga-Sutra* of Patanjali. This short text, together with its commentaries, makes up Classical Yoga, also known as *yoga-darshana* or the philosophical system of Yoga. Many paraphrases and a few good translations of this work exist. Patanjali's text is difficult to understand in parts, because it presupposes a fair amount of knowledge about Indian thought and culture. Nevertheless, it is rewarding to plow through this scripture very carefully.

A good, if technical, translation is that by J.H. Woods, which also includes the two main Sanskrit commentaries by Vyasa and Vacaspati Mishra. I can also recommend P.N. Mukerji's translation based on the exposition by the late Swami Hariharananda Aranya. Of Pandit Usharbudh Arya's fine rendering of the *Yoga-Sutra* and Vyasa's commentary, only the first volume is as yet available. I myself have authored several books on Classical Yoga, including a translation of Patanjali's aphorisms.

Many Sanskrit commentaries have been written on the *Yoga-Sutra*. These are all exceedingly technical. However, serious students may want to know that translations of two important Sanskrit commentaries, or at least of parts of them, are at long last available in English: the *Yoga-Varttika* of Vijnana Bhikshu and the *Yoga-Bhashya-Vivarana* of Shankara. The latter work is particularly fascinating, since it apparently was composed by the same Shankara who, later, became the great proponent of Advaita Vedanta.

Post-Classical Yoga is embodied in a great many works. First there are the texts of *hatha-yoga*, such as the *Hatha-Yoga-Pradipika*, the *Gheranda-Samhita*, the *Shiva-Samhita*, the *Goraksha-Samhita*, the *Hatha-Ratnavali*, the *Yoga-Bija*, the *Yoga-Shastra* of Dattatreya, the *Sat-Karma-Samgraha*, and the *Shiva-Svarodaya*. Then there are the so-called *Yoga-Upanishads*, most of which were composed after 1000 A.D. These are all available in varyingly reliable translations. The Adyar Library edition contains no fewer than twenty texts.

To round out your study you also should look at sections of the bulky but inspiring *Yoga-Vasishtha* or read through its traditional abridgment, the *Laghu-Yoga-Vasishtha*. In addition, your study of

Yoga would be incomplete without also paying attention to the major *Puranas* and *Tantras,* as well as the *Moksha-Dharma* of the *Mahabharata* epic.

At least read the *Bhagavata-Purana,* which is a detailed (mythological) account of the birth, life, and death of the God-man Krishna, with many wonderful and inspiring stories of yogins and ascetics. This magnificent work contains the *Uddhava-Gita,* Krishna's final esoteric instruction to Sage Uddhava.

Among the *Tantras,* of which only a few have been translated, you should definitely read the *Kula-Arnava-Tantra.* I have discussed many of these works in more detail in my book *Yoga: The Technology of Ecstasy.* It will give you a sense of the literary treasures waiting to be discovered and enjoyed by the serious Yoga student.

To encounter the world of Yoga through its literature will challenge you in many ways. The texts are often difficult to comprehend and demand serious concentration and perseverance. You do not have to become a scholar, yet your study will show you what it takes to be a real *yogin* and what tools Yoga puts at your disposal. It also will further your self-understanding and strengthen your commitment to practice.

BIBLIOGRAPHIC REFERENCES

I. General:

M. Eliade, *Yoga: Immortality and Freedom.* Princeton: Princeton University Press, 1973.

M. Eliade, *Patanjali and Yoga.* New York: Schocken Books, 1975.

G. Feuerstein, *Yoga: The Technology of Ecstasy.* Los Angeles: J.P. Tarcher, 1989.

G. Feuerstein, *Encyclopedic Dictionary of Yoga.* New York: Paragon House, 1990.

R.K. Rai, *Encyclopedia of Yoga.* Varanasi, India: Prachya Prakashan, 1975.

J. Varenne, *Yoga and the Hindu Tradition.* Chicago, IL: University of Chicago Press, 1976.

II. *Upanishads*:

T.R.S. Ayyangar, *The Yoga Upanisads*. Adyar, India: Adyar Library, 1952.

P. Deussen, *Philosophy of the Upanishads*. New York: Dover Publications,1966.

P. Deussen, *Sixty Upanishads*. Mystic, CT.: Verry, Lawrence & Co., 1980. 2 vols.

R.E. Hume, *The Thirteen Principal Upanishads*. Oxford, England: Oxford University Press, 1971.

K. Prem, *The Yoga of the Kathopanishad*. London: Watkins, 1955.

S. Radhakrishnan, *The Principal Upanisads*. Atlantic Highlands, NJ: Humanities Press, 1978.

III. *Bhagavad-Gita*:

S. Aurobindo, *Essays on the Gita*. Pondicherry, India: Auromere, 1979.

G. Feuerstein, *Introduction to the Bhagavad-Gita*. Wheaton, IL: Quest Books, 1983.

K. Prem, *The Yoga of the Bhagavat Gita*. Harmondsworth, England: Penguin Books, 1973.

S. Radhakrishnan, *The Bhagavadgita*. San Francisco: Harper & Row, n.d.

R.C. Zaehner, *The Bhagavad-Gita*. Oxford, England: Oxford University Press, 1969.

IV. *Mahabharata*:

W. Buck, *Mahabharata*. Berkeley, CA: University of California Press, 1973. [A condensed retelling]

M.N. Dutt, *A Prose English Translation of the Mahabharata*. Calcutta, India: H.C. Dass, 1895-1905. 8 vols.

F. Edgerton, *The Beginnings of Indian Philosophy*. London: Allen & Unwin, 1965.

V. *Yoga-Sutra* and its Commentaries:

H. Aranya, *Yoga Philosophy of Patanjali*. Transl. by P.N. Mukerji. Calcutta: University of Calcutta, 1977.

U. Arya, *Yoga-Sutras of Patanjali with the Exposition of Vyasa: A Translation and Commentary—Volume I: Samadhi-Pada*. Honesdale, PA: Himalayan International Institute, 1986.

G. Feuerstein, *The Yoga-Sutra of Patanjali: A New Translation and Commentary*. Rochester, VT: Inner Traditions International, 1989.

G. Feuerstein, *The Philosophy of Classical Yoga*. Manchester, England: Manchester University Press, 1981.

T. Leggett, *The Complete Commentary by Sankara on the Yoga Sutras: A Full Translation of the Newly Discovered Text*. London and New York: Kegan Paul International, 1990.

T.S. Rukmani, *Yogavarttika of Vijnanabhiksu*. New Delhi: Munshiram Manoharlal, 1981, 1983, 1987, 1989. 4 vols.

J.H. Woods, *Yoga System of Patanjali*. New Delhi: Motilal Banarsidass, 1977. [Includes translations of the *Yoga-Bhashya* and the *Tattva-Vaisharadi* commentaries]

VI. *Tantras, Puranas, Yoga-Vasishtha*:

K. Narayanaswamy Aiyer, *Laghu-Yoga-Vasistha*. Madras, India: Adyar Library and Research Center, 1975.

A. Avalon, *Shakti and Shakta*. New York: Dover Publications, 1978.

V.L. Mitra, *The Yoga-Vasishtha-Maharamayana*. Varanasi, India: Bharatiya Publishing House, 1976. 4 vols.

M.P. Pandit, *The Kularnava Tantra*. Madras, India: Ganesh, 1973.

Swami Kuvalayananda and Swami Digambarji, *Vasistha Samhita: Yoga Kanda*. Lonavla, India: Kaivalyadhama, 1969.

Swami Madhavananda, *Uddhava Gita*. Calcutta, India: Advaita Ashrama, 1971.

Swami Venkatesananda, *The Concise Yoga Vasistha*. Albany, NY: State University of New York Press, 1984.

VII. *Hatha-Yoga* Scriptures:

A. Avalon, *The Serpent Power*. New York: Dover Publications, 1974.

B.M. Awasthi, *Yoga Bija*. Delhi: Swami Keshwananda Yoga Institute, n.d.

B.M. Awasthi and A. Sharma, *Yoga Sastra of Dattatreya*. Delhi: Swami Keshawananda Yoga Institute, 1985.

R.G. Harshe, *Satkarmasangrahah*. Lonavla, India: Kaivalyadhama, 1970.

S. Iyangar, *The Hathayogapradipika of Svatmarama*. Madras, India: Adyar Library and Research Center, 1972.

R.K. Rai, *Shiva Svarodaya*. Varanasi, India: Prachya Parakashan, 1980.

M.V. Reddy, *Hatharatnavali*. Arthamuru, India: M. Ramakrishna Reddy, 1982.

Swami Digambarji and M.L. Gharote, *Gheranda Samhita*. Lonavla, India: Kaivalyadhama, 1978.

Swami Digambarji and R. Kokaje, *Hathayogapradipika of Svatmarama*. Lonavla, India: Kaivalyadhama, 1970.

Swami Kuvalayananda and S.A. Shukla, *Goraksasatakam*. Lonavla, India: Kaivalyadhama, 1958.

S.C. Vasu, The Gheranda Samhita: *A Treatise on Hatha Yoga*. London: Theosophical Publishing House, 1976.

S.C. Vasu, *The Siva Samhita*. New Delhi: Oriental Books Reprint Corp., 1975.

5

SCIENCE STUDIES YOGA

1. OVERVIEW

Western science has grown out of magic and alchemy, though scientists seldom care to acknowledge this historical truth or ponder its implications. In fact, science has reached its present preeminence by rejecting its own past, condemning it as mythology. Undoubtedly, the success of science, double-edged as it has proven to be, has been due to its rejection of traditional (religious) authority. But—as has become clear especially in the last eighty years—in following the authority of experiment and logic, science has not only opened up new vistas but also closed a good many doors upon reality.

In particular, in its pursuit of absolute objectivity, science has created its own elaborate mythology. Although anxious to hold apart facts from values, scientists have in actuality elevated science to the level of a philosophy or, more accurately, an ideology with its own distinct set of values. When we think of science today, we do not primarily think of a practical approach to gathering information but an overarching model of the universe: Modern science is perpetuating itself as *scientism*.

In rejecting its own "mythological" past, science also had to reject the human psyche and the entire dimension of the spirit. Indeed, for an entire generation, scientists—who were known as behaviorists—indulged in the absurd habit of striking the word "consciousness" from their vocabulary. Consciousness, they said, is not measurable and therefore it does not exist.

This positivist position was subsequently completely undermined by the discoveries of quantum physics, which showed that the observing consciousness is somehow implicated in the realities it observes. In effect, this new discipline, more than any other, wreaked havoc with the established scientific paradigm. For it demonstrated that Nature is, after all, not "rational" but an unbelievably complex and multidimensional field of interacting forces that ultimately defies understanding.

This opened a sluice through which the wisdom of the East could flow once again into our ailing Western civilization, enriching and enlivening it. We have to say "once again," because many of the things we value and in which we take pride have their origins in the East: writing, mathematics, astronomy, chronometry, the theatrical arts, and even biofeedback therapy.

This massive shift in the materialistic paradigm that has dominated our Euro-American civilization for more than two hundred years is the background against which we must understand the contemporary interest in the ideas and practices of Yoga. In the face of the breakdown of scientistic ideology, scientists are today more willing to look at worldviews such as Yoga or Vedanta that entertain beliefs and notions contradicting the materialistic-mechanistic paradigm. In Yoga, they are encountering a rich and mature "counter-technology" that is based on centuries-long exploration of the inner or psychic cosmos.

The earliest scientific interest in Yoga was piqued by some of the more spectacular yogic feats, notably live burials, which are reasonably well documented. Though these are more fakiristic techniques than yogic practices, the curiosity of the medical profession was appropriately roused, contributing to the feeling that Yoga deserved closer study.

Renewed interest in pit burials emerged in the 1950s. According to one report, ten thousand people witnessed the burial of a *yogin* who stayed under ground for sixty-two hours. When he emerged from the pit, he was examined by a physician who, not surprisingly, found a drastic reduction in the rate of metabolism, suggesting a "hibernation effect." Control of the body's metabolism is a stable feature of yogic techniques.

At the turn of the century, with the rise of psychiatry, a number of physicians confessed to being intrigued by the apparent ability of *yogins* to influence the autonomic nervous system. Among the first medical doctors to look into Yoga was the German physician

J. H. Schultz, who later invented Autogenic Training, which has been hailed as the Western equivalent to Indian Yoga. However, Schultz's method derived from his extensive experimentation with hypnosis during the period from 1905 to 1920 rather than, as is often assumed, from his acquaintance with Yoga.

In the fourth edition of his work, Schultz observed that "from a medical-psychological viewpoint, Yoga appears to have originally sprung from a gigantic, even cosmic hypochondria,"[1] because every exercise is presented as an avenue to immortality. This is of course an unfortunate misrepresentation of Yoga, but it did not prevent Schultz from being impressed with this age-old tradition. "When one omits," he admitted, "all the phantastic accessories, the profundity and subtlety of Yoga are surprising."[2] True to the positivistic spirit of his day, Schultz expressed his confidence that, in due course, scientists would discover the "real content" of Yoga, hidden beneath what he considered to be useless accretions. He compared this situation to the creation of rational hypnotherapy out of the earlier mystical magnetism.

Schultz agreed with the German historian of religion Friedrich Heiler that Yoga is primarily a "mystical psycho-technology" that is directed toward a spiritual goal. In contrast to this, he characterized his Autogenic Training as a "biological-rational technology having the goal of autonomous organismic personality development."[3] Nevertheless, he admitted that there are many parallels between the two approaches, not least the insistence on proper guidance by an expert. As he put it, "Autogenic Training and Yoga as well as all cognate serious endeavors actually stand on the same ever-young shores."[4]

While there is much in the Yoga tradition, especially *hatha-yoga*, that appears to belong to the realm of confabulation, it would be quite wrong to "de-mythologize" Yoga. For, we would be left with an empty shell. Instead, we should study Yoga from within, as practitioners rather than cool, "objective" observers. So long as we judge from the outside we can see only what our preconceived ("rational") categories permit us to see.

For instance, we can measure skin response, brain waves, or heartbeat on yogic subjects, but this tells us very little about *how* they accomplish their extraordinary states or what they *mean* to them in the larger context of life. Only as practitioners can we allow the wisdom and power of Yoga to unfold before our eyes without interfering with the process, and then perhaps what appears as fiction and fantasy from the outside will be found to have experiential value after all.

In the 1920s and 1930s, the principal interest in Yoga was from the viewpoint of psychology and psychotherapy. The medical journals in Europe and the United States started to carry papers on the clinical effects of meditation, though another four decades had to pass before this line of research was pursued more seriously. The main reason for this later development was undoubtedly the greater availability of meditators—thanks to the popularity of "Transcendental Meditation" as taught by Maharishi Mahesh Yogi.

The earliest scientific studies on the physiological effects of Yoga were those conducted by the French cardiologist Thérèse Brosse. In 1935, she traveled to India to take EKG recordings on subjects who were varyingly skilled in different forms of Yoga. This study initiated a line of investigation that was continued more vigorously from the 1960s onward.

Brosse's work also encouraged the controlled study of brain waves in meditative and other states, starting in the mid-1950s. This research was pioneered by N. N. Das (an Indian physician) and H. Gastaut (a French doctor), and it set the stage for a good many further experiments.

What all these studies succeeded in demonstrating to one degree or another is that "there is something to Yoga." Proficient *yogins* or meditators were found to be able to control many bodily processes that had previously been thought to be entirely autonomous. This also lent credibility to many of the otherwise strange explanations and concepts of Yoga, and today some of the claims that have been made by Self-realized adepts through the centuries appear far less outlandish than they once seemed.

2. MEDICAL STUDIES ON *HATHA-YOGA* PRACTICES

The first laboratory dedicated to the empirical study of Yoga was founded in 1924 by Swami Kuvalayananda at Lonavla in South India.

Six years earlier, Shri Yogendra had founded his Yoga Institute of Bombay, but he did not become interested in the medical aspect of Yoga until the mid-1930s. Both organizations have amassed considerable data in the interim period, and their pioneering work has been augmented by hundreds of independent projects—particularly during the past twenty years. A number of studies have been sponsored by the All-India Institute of Mental Health and, in the United States, by the Menninger Foundation (Topeka, Kansas) and the Himalayan International Institute of Yoga Science and Philosophy (Honesdale, Pennsylvania). The latter organization is headed by Swami Rama, a *yogin* who has demonstrated astonishing control over his nervous system.

James Funderburk, a professor of mathematics and student of Swami Rama, has surveyed some of the available research data in his book *Science Studies Yoga,* which, among other things, reveals the following:

1. The practice of postures (*asana*) improves the relaxation of muscles and significantly increases flexibility, especially of the vertebral joints. The principal purpose of the postures is to prepare the body for the meditative disciplines of *raja-yoga.* James Funderburk remarked: "In view of the breadth and subtlety of such effects one can only wonder at the level of sophistication in knowledge of human physiology that gave birth to the development of the system of asanas." [5]

2. The practice of *hatha-yoga,* though not specifically designed to enhance fitness as measured on both male and female athletes, improves all-round bodily fitness.

3. The different techniques of *hatha-yoga,* notably breath control (*pranayama*), improve cardiovascular efficiency. After only a six-week period, practitioners were found to have a lower basal heart rate. Particularly, the practice of the "corpse posture" (*shava-asana*) was found to lower the heart rate by about ten beats per minute, after only fifteen minutes of practice.

4. The different "locks" (*bandha*), especially the abdominal lock (*uddiyana-bandha*), produce considerable "sub-atmospheric" pressure in the esophagus, stomach, colon, and bladder. This has been shown to have long-term beneficial effects by stimulating the colon and liver.

5. The regular practice of the inverted postures, such as the headstand

and shoulderstand, improves the peripheral blood flow; the increased blood flow to the neck is helpful in balancing the activity of the thyroid gland, which is important for regulating the body's metabolism. One subject, Swami Rama, demonstrated the high degree to which blood flow can be controlled by the mind: He produced a temperature difference of ten degrees Celsius in a small area of his right hand.

6. Regular practice of *hatha-yoga* has been found to decrease the systolic blood pressure, and this fact has been put to advantage in the treatment of hypertensive patients.

7. After a period of only six weeks of daily *hatha-yoga* practice, it was found that blood samples contained a statistically significant increase of red blood cells and hemoglobin. Other positive changes in blood chemistry have also been reported, including decreases in serum and plasma cholesterol and blood sugar.

8. Daily practice of breathing exercises has been shown to lead, after several months, to positive changes in the basal breath rate—by as much as five breaths per minute, and more. The basal rate of non-practitioners averages around twenty-three breaths per minute, whereas for experienced Yoga practitioners it has been found to average as low as ten.

9. Regular breath control also increases the time for which the breath can be held. One study has shown an average increase of twelve seconds, after only a six-week period. Also, the amount of air that a person can expel after maximal inhalation was found to be increased after several months of practice.

10. Regular *hatha-yoga* practice was demonstrated to stimulate the hormonal secretions of the body.

11. Daily practice of *hatha-yoga* enhances the functioning of the parasympathetic nervous system, which is tied in with the ability to relax at will. Particularly breath control has been found to greatly increase skin resistance. In other words, it induces deep muscular relaxation, though without drowsiness or sleep.

Some of the research done simply translates into medical terminology what common sense would expect, and may tell us no more than, say, that regular breathing exercises increase our lung capacity and strengthen the heart muscle. But the scientific method is a laborious process of assembling bits of information, piece by piece. Sometimes it discovers the unexpected or reveals rich connections between otherwise quite obvious facts. The study of the physiological effects of *hatha-yoga* is still in its infancy, and we can look forward to a host of other exciting discoveries, especially as and when medical science develops new approaches that are in consonance with a nonmaterialistic paradigm.

3. THE PHYSIOLOGY OF MEDITATION AND HIGHER STATES OF CONSCIOUSNESS

Body and mind are two aspects of a single functional system that extends far beyond the boundary of the skin. Availing himself of the great insights of the new paradigm, the American internist Larry Dossey sees the human body as part of what he calls the larger *biodance*:

> It is not only our genes that renew themselves. The entire body participates in this astonishing dynamism . . . Our replacement parts come in constant flow from the earth itself . . . *Biodance*—the endless exchange of the elements of living things with the earth itself—proceeds silently, giving us no hint that it is happening. It is a dervish dance, animated and purposeful and disciplined; and it is a dance in which every living organism participates . . . A strictly bounded body does not exist. The concept of a physical I that is fixed in space and that endures in time is at odds with our knowledge that living structures are richly connected with the world around them. Our roots go deep; we are anchored in the stars. [6]

Given that body and mind form a single pattern, it is appropriate to want to understand the physiological dimension of "higher" processes in consciousness, such as meditation and ecstasy (*samadhi*). Of course, the physiological data do not *necessarily* tell us anything useful about the subjective spiritual aspects of the experiences. At best, the research findings can suggest to us that these higher states transcend their material, somatic correlates.

For instance, when Swami Rama was tested at the Menninger Foundation, he appeared to be in a state of deep sleep according to the electroencephalographic and other evidence; yet upon "waking," he recalled environmental information more accurately than the experimenters who had, by common definition, been awake during the experiment. Nonetheless, physiological research can bring light to certain issues, providing it does not seek to monopolize the truth.

On the mistaken materialistic assumption that mental states are generated by the brain, researchers have—since the mid-1950s—endeavored to record the effects of meditation on the electrical output of the brain. The first experiments of this type were undertaken by N. N. Das and H. Gastaut on practitioners of *kriya-yoga*. This Yoga practice involves the controlled guidance of the body's bio-energy (*kundalini-shakti*) to the *ajna-cakra*, the psychospiritual locus between and behind the eyebrows. This produces an inner light, which is then made the focus of attention, leading to further photistic experiences in meditation. This research team also investigated the physiological effect of meditation on the heart and other muscles.

What Das and Gastaut found was that their meditating subjects showed an accelerated alpha rhythm accompanied by a decrease in amplitude. In addition, they recorded pronounced beta waves during states that were subsequently reported to have been ecstasy.

To appreciate what this means, we should note that brain research has identified four major wave forms on the basis of their frequencies (measured in Hertz, or cycles per second), *viz.*, (1) beta (13–30 Hz.), (2) alpha (8–13 Hz.), (3) theta (4–7 Hz.), and (4) delta (0.5–4 Hz.). The beta rhythm is typical of our ordinary waking life, when we are alert to the outside world. Alpha waves kick in when we close our eyes and enter a more relaxed state. Theta waves are associated with drowsiness, the state in between waking and sleeping, whereas delta waves are a sign of deep sleep.

Experiments on Zen practitioners have shown that alpha waves can be produced even when the eyes are open, providing a relaxed inner state is created. Swami Rama, who produced the entire spectrum of brain waves at will, achieved the alpha frequency simply by picturing a cloudless blue sky.

Das' and Gastaut's pioneering efforts were followed several years later by the research projects of M.A. Wenger, B.K. Bagchi, and B.K. Anand. Their studies partly confirmed the earlier findings. However, their subjects did not generate beta waves. At first it was thought that the earlier experiments had been faulty, but as EEG research on meditative and ecstatic states continued, it became clear that different types of meditation are associated with different brain waves.

Wenger's team complained that they were able to find only a few suitable subjects. This changed with the immense popularity of Transcendental Meditation in the 1970s. It was Robert Keith Wallace who first mapped the physiological effects of TM. His discoveries encouraged him to propose enthusiastically that the psychophysiological state of TM should be regarded as a "fourth state" in addition to waking, dreaming, and sleeping.

The most comprehensive EEG studies of TM are those by J. P. Banquet in 1972 and 1973. Banquet, a neurologist, used subjects who had been meditating for at least two years. What he found was that they produced EEG patterns that included not only the usual accelerated alpha waves but also theta and even delta rhythms, while yet reporting subjective states of awakeness.

Writing in 1976, at a time when some five hundred thousand Americans were practicing TM, Harold H. Bloomfield *et al.* hailed TM as "a major discovery in the technology of human integration."[7] While the regular practice of TM has undoubtedly beneficial effects, some of the more sweeping claims have meanwhile come under scrutiny.

Several studies revealed that during the state of deepest meditation and ecstasy, the subjects were found insensitive to painful stimuli (such as intense light, pin pricks, etc.), while high-frequency waves, including beta waves, were recorded from all EEG channels. Today medical researchers must accept that the human mind can exercise considerable control over the autonomic nervous system, and that even quite ordinary people, with a modicum of training in biofeedback, can accomplish remarkable feats of this kind. Thus, biofeedback has been used successfully in connection with tension headaches, high blood pressure, and even epilepsy.

One of the most fascinating discoveries of EEG research on meditators is that, in higher states of consciousness, there is a distinct synchronization of brain waves. In these synchronized states even the beta rhythm can appear in an integrated fashion, without suggesting a disruption of the subjectively experienced condition of meditation. For instance, at the Menninger Foundation, Swami Rama created delta frequencies at will, and the other three rhythms continued to be registered. Synchronization indicates a condition of organismic balance, which reminds one of the definition in the *Bhagavad-Gita* (II.48) that "Yoga is balance."

This finding is also substantially borne out by other physiological research on meditation, such as its effects on the muscular, circulatory, respiratory, and endocrine systems. Meditators have been found to overcome the most devastating syndrome of our era, which is "time sickness."

M. Friedman and R. H. Rosenman introduced the helpful distinction between "Type A" and "Type B" personalities.[8] The former are ambitious, goal-oriented, constantly "driven," and always at odds with time. They tend to suffer from increased heart rate, respiration, and blood pressure, and elevation of adrenalin, norepinephrine, insulin, and other hormone levels. All this translates into stress, or bodily tension. Type B individuals, by contrast, are less hurried and, as a group, less likely to suffer heart attacks and other stress-related diseases.

Meditation "dilates" time, or rather our experience of it. During meditation, we step momentarily out of the flux of events, allowing our body-mind to resonate with life at a different level, without the intrusion of our own psychic programs. Regular practice of meditation trains us in that "natural" attitude, which effects permanent changes in our body-mind.

Phil Nuernberger, a physician and a student of Swami Rama, summarized the research to date in the following words:

> When compared to others who do not practice meditation, or to their own state before they began to meditate, those who consistently practice meditation are healthier, happier, and more effective human beings. Clinical experience, scientific research, and the experience of the layperson all point to one and the same conclusion: the consistent practice of meditation is probably the most important and effective self-help tool available today for personal health and effectiveness. It is also clear that under the guidance of a competent instructor, meditation can be safely and successfully practiced by almost anyone, excluding the fanatic or the psychotic, without fear of harmful side-effects.[9]

While the benefit of regular meditation practice is beyond dispute, we must not forget that within the framework of traditional Yoga, meditation is not so much a therapeutic device as one of the steps toward Self-realization. Nuernberger acknowledged this when he wrote:

When, through meditation, we come to experience directly our true spiritual identity, the personality with all its peaks and valleys no longer exerts a claim. We experience an inner calm and tranquility, a center that is secure and free of conflict . . . From this center, we can consciously choose creative and fruitful actions in the world, being responsive to, but not reacting to, the ups and downs of the changing world.[10]

That meditation can entail a variety of psychological and physiological responses has been demonstrated by the above-mentioned studies of Das and Gastaut. It appears that the meditative state generated by *kundalini-yoga* differs markedly from other forms of meditation in that it is far more dynamic. The symptoms of an "awakened" psychospiritual energy of the *kundalini* can be spectacular and even alarming, especially when the arousal of this super-energy occurs spontaneously and without adequate preparation and guidance. Gopi Krishna has given us a most vivid account of the nightmarish aspects of the *kundalini* process.

But the *kundalini* has claimed not a few "victims" also in the West. The American psychiatrist Lee Sannella, who was among the first to counsel such people, tried to unravel this rather obscure phenomenon by using the vibrational model developed by Itzhak Bentov, which distinguishes between a "physio-*kundalini*" and the *kundalini* as a spiritual phenomenon.

Bentov's model suggests that meditation sets up an electromagnetic oscillation that synchronizes the natural oscillation in the aorta, the heart, the ventricles, and the brain. This synchronized oscillation involves a sine wave of approximately seven cycles per second. According to Bentov, this rhythm corresponds to the electromagnetic frequency found in the "resonant cavity" of the earth's atmosphere. Once a meditator has reached a certain depth of meditation, he or she becomes subject to what is known as "rhythm entrainment," that is, he or she becomes locked into the frequency of our planet. This explains, for instance, why it is generally difficult to "snap out" of deep meditation at will.

Sannella, like Gopi Krishna, understands the *kundalini* as *the* evolutionary mechanism. This idea clearly goes beyond the Darwinian model of Western biology, but, as the renowned German physicist and philosopher Carl Friedrich von Weizsäcker has argued, is worthy of consideration.[11]

4. PSYCHOTHERAPY AND YOGA

Modern psychotherapy is a science-based effort to restore the individual human psyche to wholeness. It has grown out of the clinical treatment of cases that medical science was unable to help effectively. At the turn of the century, neurologists became fascinated with the dramatic symptoms of hysteria, such as insensitivity or hypersensitivity of parts of the body, and they explored hypnosis as a means of dealing with these symptoms. In trying to understand the particular suffering of hysterical patients, Sigmund Freud (1856–1939) elaborated his well-known theory and method of psychoanalysis.

In a nutshell, Freud's therapeutic system is based on the recognition that human life is largely governed by unconscious impulses—an insight shared with the Eastern liberation teachings. The human personality is, according to Freud, a tripartite system consisting of the conscious mind, the subconscious, and the unconscious. The last-mentioned is the seat of the fundamental energy that drives the entire system. That energy is called *libido* and is primarily sexual in nature. The parallels to the Indian idea of the *kundalini,* which is a form of the universal life-force (*prana*), have often been pointed out.

Freud and his followers believe that all mental problems, insofar as they do not have a direct physical origin (such as brain damage), are the result of a faulty adaptation of the libido, such as its conversion into sexual obsessions or religious fanaticism. The task of psychoanalysis—Freud's particular system of psychotherapy—is to repair existing maladaptations and thus to free the libido for more healthy expressions such as, for instance, artistic creativity.

Freud's work contributed immeasurably to the recognition that the ego and the rational mind are rather fragile developments in contrast with the background of the vast irrational forces of the unconscious. For him, religion was one of the "civilized" attempts to deal with these chaotic forces. Freud, who was steeped in the positivistic tradition of the nineteenth century, nevertheless saw religion as an illusory, if mostly benign, compensatory mechanism. Freud knew very little about Yoga and Eastern philosophies, but this did not prevent him from passing summary judgement on them.[12]

The book *Mystical Experience* by the Israeli philosopher Ben-Ami Scharfstein includes a chapter on "Freud's Psychoanalysis and Patanjali's Yoga." In this essay, Scharfstein argues that the aims of these two systems are as far apart as the cultural environment in which they were created. But he sees certain methodological parallels between them.

First, he points out, both Freud and Patanjali insist on the drivenness of the human being: We are normally governed by our passions or instincts, notably the will to survive as an individual. Both Freud and Patanjali assume that the human psyche includes a function that the former called "repression," by which we forget our own past experience. Yet, that past is, for both, a powerfully dynamic ingredient of our present adaptation to life.

For both Freud and Patanjali, our redemption lies in our reaching back into our own past, as it has sedimented in the unconscious. Once we have understood our own psychic program, we can begin to institute countermeasures. Self-observation is the key in either approach. However, whereas the psychoanalyst seeks to restore the patient suffering from neurosis or psychosis to balanced functioning in the world, based on a feeling of having come to terms with his or her own existence in the world, the teacher (*guru*) seeks to awaken the disciple to a different reality altogether.

Scharfstein rightly observes that the *yogin*'s objective is to go beyond his attachment to the world, beyond his fixation and dependence on external things. He reads this, in psychoanalytic jargon, as a movement toward *depersonalization*. However, Scharfstein notes that the *yogin*'s "depersonalization" is a happy affair, whereas the depersonalization of the ordinary neurotic plunges him or her into painful meaninglessness and the desperate feeling of being out of touch with reality. The Yoga practitioner's spiritual work moves him or her effectively beyond his or her own conditioning. Yet Scharfstein makes the following criticism:

> Being Western, I cannot help feeling that the accomplishment of the Yogin, even the one who practises the most philosophical and contemplative type of Yoga, the kind which has been described here, is too selfish and too nourished on fantasies. The serious Yogin has

substantial insight and great discipline, but he uses insight and discipline to remain self-enclosed. Freud's well-known contrast of the basic forces of Eros [the will to live] and Thanatos [the will to die] is congenial to Indian thought, but while Freud chooses Eros, the Yogin chooses Thanatos, or timelessness, isolation, and quiescence, which we call simply death. [13]

This critique of Yoga ignores the important fact that even Patanjali, who avows a particularly stringent form of world-renunciation, lists compassion (*karuna*) among the virtues to be cultivated by the *yogin*. However, Scharfstein is correct in highlighting the infelicitous tendency in mystical circles to downplay ordinary reality and its concerns. Yet, Scharfstein is wrong in asserting that if mysticism ever came to "dominate" the world, "it would impoverish mankind materially, intellectually, and spiritually." [14]

Freud's student and erstwhile collaborator Carl Gustav Jung (1875–1962) sought to do better justice to the universal religious or spiritual impulse. His clinical experience had taught him that neurotics are suffering from an existential (religious) crisis, and that psychic wholeness is restored only when the individual has found his or her true relationship to the larger life. Thus, Jungian therapy serves as a Western counterpart to the Eastern liberation teachings. Given Jung's general orientation, it is understandable that he should have made extensive use of the wisdom found in alchemy, occultism, and such Eastern traditions as Taoism and *kundalini-yoga*.

Nevertheless, as psychotherapist Hans Jacobs and others have shown, Jung never really understood the Eastern liberation schools—notwithstanding the fact that he wrote copiously about them. [15] This failure is epitomized in his mistaken assumption that the condition of ecstasy (*samadhi*) is nothing but a meaningless dream state. [16] Apparently, Jung could not conceive of a state of awareness that transcended the ego and yet did not sink into unconsciousness. Even though he spoke frequently of the Self, he did not mean the transcendental Self, as revealed in yogic Self-realization, but an "archetype" of psychic experience. As Swami Akhilananda remarked:

Professor Jung seems to conclude that the superconscious experiences are "vast but dim" without any understanding of them. Any man who has had these realizations will laugh at such conclusions.

Patanjali, Swami Vivekananda, and Swami Brahmananda give just the opposite point of view. They make it clear that *samadhi,* or the superconscious state, is vivid and definite. [17]

A less biased and far more encouraging appraisal of Yoga than Jung's was given by the British psychoanalyst Geraldine Coster, who wrote:

> That yoga in its traditional forms is essentially an eastern practice unsuited to western life and temperament I am prepared to admit . . . Nevertheless, I am convinced that the ideas on which yoga is based are universally true for mankind, and that we have in the yoga sutras a body of material which we could investigate and use with infinite advantage. [18]

Coster argued that Yoga is just as practical as analytical therapy, and she also expressed her conviction that the *Yoga-Sutra* of Patanjali contains the information sought by the most advanced psychotherapists of her day.

Coster wrote her book more than fifty years ago. Meanwhile psychotherapy has undergone a quiet revolution, leading to the emergence of humanistic psychology and then transpersonal psychology—the "third" and "fourth force," respectively. Building on the great insights of Freud and Jung, these new psychologies have taken cognizance of the fact that human well-being is not confined to smooth physical and mental functioning as part of the social organism.

Humanistic psychologists introduced a wider concept of wholeness, which includes what Abraham Maslow—the doyen of the third force—called "self-actualization." Transpersonal psychology went a step further, acknowledging that human beings are not only capable of realizing their psychological potential but also of transcending themselves. Again it was Maslow who pointed the way when, toward the end of his life, he regarded self-transcendence as one of the biologically anchored needs. Today transpersonal psychology represents the leading edge in the encounter between East and West. In the words of Roger Walsh and Frances Vaughan:

> The goals of transpersonal therapy include both traditional ones such as symptom relief and behavior change, and where appropriate, optimal work at the transpersonal level . . . In addition to working through

psychodynamic processes, the therapist aims to assist the client in disidentifying from and transcending psychodynamic issues. . . .

Transpersonal therapeutic techniques include both Eastern and Western methods for working with consciousness. Various forms of meditation and yoga may be added to more conventional techniques. [19]

The problem with the transpersonal approach is that therapists are therapists and not *yogins,* and so their recommendations may arguably not always be adequately informed. A group of medical practitioners who have also undergone extensive yogic "training" is the team around Swami Rama. The book *Yoga and Psychotherapy,* co-authored by Swami Rama, embodies perhaps the most integrated application of Yoga in psychotherapy so far.

5. PARAPSYCHOLOGICAL RESEARCH

Paranormal phenomena do not fit into the ruling paradigm of scientific materialism, and hence they are either ignored or explained away. The hostility of the scientific establishment toward the young discipline of parapsychology is well known. Yet, again and again science encounters so-called psychic phenomena that cannot be adequately accounted for by the usual labels of "hallucination," "delusion," "perceptual error," "superstition," or "deliberate deception."

Paranormal abilities and occurrences are what one might call a "universal constant" of the world's psychospiritual traditions. Unless we assume that millions of people in hundreds of different cultures over thousands of years have all been subject to mass hypnosis, fraud, or wishful thinking, we must at least be willing to look at the available evidence. What we are in fact presented with is a considerable amount of data that are strongly suggestive of a paranormal order of events.

Parapsychology has come a long way since the founding of the Society for Psychical Research in England in 1882 and its American counterpart in Boston three years later. The massive statistical research by J.B. Rhine at Duke University from the 1930s to the 1950s, the work of Ian Stevenson at the University of Virginia Medical School since the late 1960s, the *psi* projects at the Stanford Research

Institute and the Maimonides Medical Center—all have demonstrated that paranormal phenomena need to be taken seriously.

Yoga is founded on an understanding of the universe as a multidimensional psychophysical process rather than a one-dimensional materialistic structure. From the beginning, the *yogin* has been celebrated and possibly feared by the popular mind as a magician and worker of miracles. Therefore it should not come as a surprise that Patanjali devoted an entire chapter of his *Yoga-Sutra* to techniques for cultivating paranormal powers. The method he recommended is known as *samyama* or "constraint," which is the combined practice of concentration, meditation, and ecstasy with regard to the same object.

This method yields superknowledge (*prajna*) and is recognized as a form of valid cognition by most other schools of Indian philosophy. It is also known as *yogi-pratyaksha* or "yogic perception." There is no psychic phenomenon that is not found in the literature of Yoga. But the most spectacular claims revolve around the tradition of the set of eight major paranormal powers (*maha-siddhi*). These are hinted at by Patanjali in aphorism III.45, and his commentator Vyasa supplies the following list:

(1) miniaturization (*animan*) of the body;

(2) magnification (*mahiman*) of the body;

(3) levitation (*laghiman*);

(4) extension (*prapti*), i.e., the ability to "touch the moon with the fingertips";

(5) irresistible will (*prakamya*), i.e., the ability to defy the properties of the material elements, such as the ability to move through earth as if it were water;

(6) mastery (*vashitva*), i.e., dominion over material Nature;

(7) lordship (*ishitritva*), i.e., supremacy over body and mind;

(8) fulfillment of desires (*kama-avasayitva*), i.e., the power of determining events according to one's desires, such as turning poison into nectar.

These eight *siddhis* are also called the "lordly powers" (*aishvarya*), because they simulate the abilities of the Creator (*ishvara*). Other schools of Yoga know of different lists, though the powers specified are all equally astonishing.

What are we to make of these abilities? Are they merely the products of a lively fantasy triggered by too much solitary introspection? Or are they manifestations of a psychic dimension of reality that science still needs to discover? Over the centuries, all kinds of anecdotal reports have come down to us of the uncommon powers of *yogins* and psychic phenomena witnessed in their company.

For instance, Kamil V. Zvelebil, a respected scholar of the Tamil language and culture, related how one of his Siddha "informants" succeeded in producing, "out of apparent nothing, a very substantial chunk of matter," which he reluctantly explained as "a kind of game with anti-matter." [20] Did the good professor succumb to a sleight of hand or hypnotic suggestion? Or, ruling out that he was merely lying, did he really witness a paranormal event? The same questions can be asked of some of the stories found in the autobiographical works of Swami Yogananda [21] and Swami Rama, [22] as well as the biography of the great twentieth-century ascetic Tapasviji Maharaj. [23] In fact, the literature on saints and sages of whatever persuasion or period is replete with accounts that involve paranormal occurrences.

We find that Swami Rama, for one, is not uncritical toward such phenomena, while still insisting that they can be authentic. He writes:

> Later I realized that mostly such phenomena are tricks. Wherever they are found to be genuine, they are black magic. Spirituality has nothing to do with these miracles. . . . One person in millions does indeed have *siddhis*, but I have found that such people are often greedy, egotistical and ignorant. The path of enlightenment is different from the intentional cultivation of powers. The miracles performed by Buddha, Christ and other great sages were spontaneous and for a purpose. They were not performed with selfish motives or to create a sensation. . . . *Siddhis* do exist, but only with adepts. [24]

In India the general attitude toward the paranormal powers is that the spiritual practitioner should completely avoid them and their display. However, Patanjali would hardly have devoted so much space to them in his *Yoga-Sutra* if he shared this view. He obviously considered the technique of ecstatic constraint (*samyama*) as a valid means of gaining extraordinary knowledge and powers.

While there is today ample evidence of the *yogins'* incredible control over bodily and mental functions that had long been thought to be outside the reach of our personal will, their claims to paranormal abilities have so far been only very scantily researched. However, the cumulative weight of the findings of parapsychological research on nonyogic subjects increasingly lends credence to many of the ideas and anecdotal reports of paranormal events and phenomena current in yogic circles.

6. SUMMARY

As we have seen, many aspects of Yoga are amenable to scientific investigation. However, certain of the claims made by *yogins* exceed either the interest or the methodological capacities of present-day science. And, finally, there are those aspects of Yoga which are intrinsically unverifiable by objective scientific means. This includes the very goal of Yoga, which is the transcendental or spiritual dimension. Thus, the Self (*atman* or *purusha*), which is by definition beyond all form and comprehension, cannot be examined under a microscope or exposed to high-energy radiation for atomic measurements. Its existence is evident solely by way of direct intuition, or enlightenment, which is a human ability that is denied by contemporary materialistic science.

Perhaps, as the scientific enterprise overcomes its inherent materialistic bias, scientists will be able to extend their repertoire to include methods capable of investigating "subtle" (*sukshma*) phenomena, which are now considered part of metaphysics. This might encourage a more tolerant attitude toward spiritual realities in general. Moreover, a duly self-critical science, which has exorcised the ghost of materialism, would then endorse the pursuit of a self-transcending life, which alone can bring us personal verification of the great Being in whom everything unfolds. At that point, science would truly have come full circle by recovering its original sacred mission, as it informed the early civilizations, particularly pharaonic Egypt. Clearly, it is of great evolutionary importance to keep the encounter between science and Yoga and other similar traditions alive.

NOTES

1. J.H. Schultz, *Das autogene Training* (Leipzig, Germany: Georg Thieme, 1940), p. 264.

2. *Ibid.*, p. 264.

3. J.H. Schultz, "Autogenes Training und Yoga," in Wilhelm Bitter, ed., *Abendländische Therapie und östliche Weisheit: Ein Tagungsbericht* (Stuttgart: Ernst Klett, 1968), p. 177.

4. *Ibid.*, p. 180.

5. J. Funderburk, *Science Studies Yoga: A Review of Physiological Data* (Glenview, IL: Himalayan International Institute, 1977), p. 15.

6. L. Dossey, *Space, Time & Medicine* (Boulder, CO; London: Shambhala, 1982), pp. 74–75.

7. H.H. Bloomfield, M.P. Cain, D.T. Jaffe, and R.B. Kory, *TM: How Meditation Can Reduce Stress* (London: Allen & Unwin, 1976), p. 6.

8. M. Friedman and H.R. Rosenman, *Type A Behavior and Your Heart* (New York: Knopf, 1974).

9. P. Nuernberger, "Mind, Meditation, and Emotions," in R.M. Ballantine, *The Theory and Practice of Meditation* (Honesdale, PA: Himalayan International Institute, 1986), p. 68.

10. *Ibid.*, p. 88.

11. See C.F. von Weizsäcker's introduction to Gopi Krishna, *Kundalini: The Biological Basis of Religion and Genius* (New Delhi: Kundalini Research and Publication Trust, 1978).

12. See, e.g., S. Freud, *Civilization and Its Discontents* (New York: W.W. Norton, 1961), p. 26.

13. B.-A. Scharfstein, *Mystical Experience* (Baltimore, MD: Penguin Books, 1974), pp. 131–132.

14. *Ibid.*, p. 174.

15. See H. Jacobs, *Western Psychotherapy and Hindu Sadhana* (London: Allen & Unwin, 1961).

16. See Jung's psychological commentary to W.Y. Evans-Wentz, *The Tibetan Book of the Great Liberation* (London/Oxford: Oxford University Press, 1968), pp. xxix–lxiv.

17. Swami Akhilananda, *Hindu Psychology: Its Meaning for the West* (London: Routledge & Sons, 1947), p. 165

18. G. Coster, *Yoga and Western Psychology: A Comparison* (London: Oxford University Press, 1934), pp. 243–245.

19. R.N. Walsh and Frances Vaughan, "A Comparison of Psychotherapies," in Roger N. Walsh and Frances Vaughan, eds., *Beyond Ego: Transpersonal Dimensions in Psychology* (Los Angeles, CA: Tarcher, 1980), p.165.

20. K.V. Zvelebil, *The Poets of the Powers* (London: Rider, 1973), p. 125.

21. See Paramahansa Yogananda, *Autobiography of a Yogi* (Los Angeles, CA: Self-Realization Fellowship, 1987).

22. See Swami Ajaya, ed., *Living with the Himalayan Masters: Spiritual Experiences of Swami Rama* (Honesdale, PA: Himalayan International Institute, 1978).

23. See Murthy, T.S. Anantha, *Maharaj: A Biography of Shriman Tapasviji Maharaj, a Mahatma Who Lived for 185 Years* (San Rafael, CA: Dawn Horse Press, 1986). With a foreword by Georg Feuerstein.

24. Swami Ajaya, *Living with the Himalayan Masters*, pp. 102–103.

BIBLIOGRAPHIC REFERENCES

[Anonymous.] *Medical & Psychological Scientific Research on Yoga & Meditation: General Effects and Possible Applications.* Peo, Denmark: Scandinavian Yoga and Meditation School, 1978.

Behanan, Kovoor, T. *Yoga: A Scientific Evaluation.* New York: Dover Publications, 1959.

Brena, Steven, F. *Yoga & Medicine: The Merging of Yogic Concepts with Modern Medical Knowledge.* New York/Baltimore: Penguin Books, 1973.

Funderburk, James, *Science Studies Yoga: A Review of Physiological Data.* Glenview, IL: Himalayan International Institute, 1977.

Maslow, Abraham H. *The Farther Reaches of Human Nature.* Harmondsworth, England: Penguin Books, 1971.

Mukherji, Gouri Shanker and Spiegelhoff, W. *Yoga und unsere Medizin.* Stuttgart, Germany: Hippokrates-Verlag, 1966.

Sachdeva, I.P. *Yoga and Depth Psychology.* Delhi: Banarsidass, 1978.

Swami Rama, Rudolph Ballentine, and Swami Ajaya, *Yoga and Psychotherapy: The Evolution of Consciousness.* Glenview, IL: Himalayan International Institute, 1976.

Watts, Alan, *Psychotherapy East and West.* New York: Pantheon Books, 1963.

Welwood, John, *The Meeting of the Ways: Explorations in East/West Psychology.* New York: Schocken Books, 1979.

Yoga Mimamsa [quarterly journal]. Lonavla, Poona, India. 1924–1935 and 1956–.

6

THE PATH OF WISDOM (JNANA-YOGA)

It is a well-established fact that subject and object are opposed to each other like light and darkness. Hence the tendency to superimpose attributes of the object onto the subject is a grave error. It is just as wrong to superimpose attributes of the subject onto the object. Yet, it is precisely from this kind of confusion between subject and object that we obtain such common statements as "I am this or that" and "this is mine." Now, in the final analysis, the subject is none other than the transcendental Self (*atman*), which can be "known" only through immediate apprehension. The object is also termed the "non-self" (*anatman*). This designation refers to the body, the senses, the mind, and the countless forms of the world. The superimposition is the same as ignorance (*avidya*). By contrast, the ascertainment of reality as it is, apart from the attributes superimposed on it, is known as gnosis (*vidya*).

The above passage is a paraphrase of the opening statement of Shankara's celebrated commentary on the *Brahma-Sutra* ("Aphorisms about the Absolute"), which is one of the literary mainstays of Vedanta metaphysics. Shankara, medieval India's best known philosopher-sage, wrote his explanatory treatise twelve hundred years ago. His explanations of the process by which we know reality are fundamental to *jnana-yoga*, the Yoga of wisdom.

This yogic path consists in the careful discrimination between the real (*sat*) and the "unreal" (*asat*). The real is the transcendental subject, or singular Self, and the unreal is everything that is experienced as "other": people, animals, trees, institutions, beliefs, abstract ideas. These make up what Shankara calls the "object" (*vishaya*), as opposed to the "subject" (*vishayin*).

Contrary to popular opinion, Shankara does *not* say that the things of the manifold world do not exist, merely that they are not finally real. They are different from what they appear to be inasmuch as, upon the event of enlightenment, they are all found to be the same Reality.

Shankara insisted that there are things to be experienced in the unenlightened state. But he also insisted that what we believe to be objective things are in truth the singular *brahman,* or Absolute. We who perceive the world as consisting of multiple independent objects are therefore committing a continuous error. We need to look more closely. At a distance a scarecrow looks like a man. When we get closer we can see we have been fooled. Shankara uses the example of the rope that is wrongly identified as a snake.

Ordinary knowledge and experience are based on a chronic separation of subject and object, as well as a certain confusion between them. That confusion is known in Vedanta as "superimposition" (*adhyasa* or *adhyaropa*), by which the true nature of the subject, the Self, is obscured. We wrongly equate the Self with the ego-personality, the empirical "I," which is merely a function of the body-mind.

Because of this primal error, we are able to constantly make statements like "I am happy," "I am sad," "I am lean," "I am in pain," "I know," "I grow," "I die," as well as "these are my children," "this belongs to me," "I have a body," and so on.

The same error is also responsible for our experiencing the object as other than what it is, namely the ultimate Reality. We think objects are external to us and that we must influence or control them in order to fulfill our deep-seated need for happiness. Thus the process of knowledge is inextricably linked with our emotional life as well as our spiritual destiny.

Jnana-yoga is an all-out effort to overcome the subject-object division by realizing the subject in its true form—as the transcendental Self, which is permanent, indivisible, and inherently blissful. *Jnana,* or gnosis, is both the goal and the medium of *jnana-yoga.*

The West knows its own form of knowledge-based Yoga, which was first strikingly formulated by Descartes. In his famous essay *Discours de la Méthode* (Discourse on Method), published in 1637, Descartes mused that "the ground of our opinions is far more custom and example than any certain knowledge."[1] But he was bent on acquiring unshakeable knowledge. His intellectual Yoga consisted in suspending prejudice and in analyzing matters so exhaustively that there is no doubt left. This strictly rational procedure is now the basis for the entire Western scientific enterprise, at least in theory.

In conceptual sophistication Shankara and Descartes are certainly on a par. However, their approaches could not be more divergent. Descartes, who represents the Western way of science, wanted absolute certainty of knowledge so that he could live a morally sound life. He saw humanity's salvation in the acquisition of more and more accurate and expansive knowledge until reality stands revealed in its nakedness.

According to Descartes, such knowledge can only be acquired through the discipline of reason. He placed little faith in the evidence of the senses or the faculty of imagination, but he implicitly trusted reason. It was in this way that he arrived at the famous Cartesian dictum: *cogito ergo sum*, "I think therefore I am." For Descartes, thought was the only means of certainty, from which one could even deduce one's own existence and the existence of everything else.

Shankara, representing the East, would have been baffled by Descartes' logic and his apparent satisfaction with a merely rational certainty. Shankara wanted an altogether different kind of certainty—the certainty of Being. In his view, Being is a self-evident fact, as obvious as sunlight, requiring no intervention of reason, and thought is a derivative of Being—even a falsification of it.

More than that, Shankara believed that conventional "knowledge" is ultimately circular, or what in philosophical jargon is called "tautological." Knowledge which is based on the split between subject and object is a matter of the mind and mental categories and not a matter of Reality. Unlike Descartes, Shankara did not think that reason furnishes us with absolute certainties. On the contrary, he held that for the most part the mind is an obstruction to the truth. Reiterating the wisdom of the ancient Hindu sages, he described the mind as the organ of doubt (*samshaya*). But doubt, for him, was not only not a desirable state but a clear indication that Being, Truth, had not yet been realized.

Shankara's position has been reaffirmed in our own century by

Sri Aurobindo, a Self-realized *yogin* who also happened to be one of modern India's greatest philosophers and poets. He observed:

> The intellect, it is said, is man's highest instrument and he must think and act according to its ideas. But this is not true; the intellect needs an inner light to guide, check and control it quite as much as the vital. There is something above the intellect which one has to discover and the intellect should be only an intermediary for the action of that source of true Knowledge. [2]

Thus, Aurobindo did not dismiss the intellect altogether. He merely sought to delimit its authority. Similarly, Shankara admitted that, at its best, knowledge (as wisdom) can at least point beyond itself. In this sense, reason is not entirely illusory or futile as an instrument of knowledge. Shankara was by no means an irrationalist. Yet he understood the limits of reason very clearly. The same can be said of Paul Brunton, a contemporary *jnana-yogin*, who wrote:

> The mistake of the mystics is to negate reasoning *prematurely*. Only after reasoning has completed its own task to the uttermost will it be psychologically right and philosophically fruitful to still it in the mystic silence. [3]

Brunton understood *jnana-yoga* as the path of "philosophic insight"—an understanding that transforms and grasps our whole being by widening our horizon beyond the ken of the ego. Philosophic insight, *jnana*, gives us a glimpse of Reality, which all at once or progressively shatters our preconceptions and connects us to our true identity, the Self. It is this connection, or communion, which gives us certainty beyond the canons of logic, dogma, and mere belief.

The absolute certainty to which Shankara aspired, and apparently had realized at a young age, visits us only when all conventional knowledge is transcended together with the knower and the known. This realization, which is synonymous with spiritual enlightenment, is the quintessence of *jnana-yoga*. It is also the core of Vedanta metaphysics, for which *jnana-yoga* is the path of realization.

Jnana-yoga is the path of insight or wisdom. Such insight, however, is not knowledge as commonly understood, but a higher or metaphysical type of illuminative knowledge, which has been called "gnosis" by some scholars. The scriptures of Vedanta distinguish between a higher knowledge, called *jnana*, and a lower knowledge, called *vijnana*. The former pertains to the organ of wisdom, or *buddhi*.[4] The latter is a product of the brain-dependent "mind," which functions as a processing plant for the input from the senses. This "lower" mind is known in the Sanskrit language as *manas*, the instrument of thought.[5]

The *buddhi* is that aspect of our being which is natively like a limpid pool—still and clear—and therefore capable of reflecting the light of the Self, the esoteric "sun." The *atman* is described as being self-luminous, whereas all finite objects, including the *buddhi*, depend for their visibility on the transcendental "light."

To employ a modern metaphor: The *atman*'s radiance is comparable to the bright light emitted by the high-powered lamp of a lighthouse. That light is reflected in the Fresnel lens surrounding the source of light; the lens corresponds to the *buddhi*. The area beyond the lighthouse is progressively darker—an image that depicts very well the dimness into which the material body and the physical world as a whole are plunged. In more literal terms, the cosmos is a fabric woven of light and darkness. Some cosmic structures (black holes) even trap light by curving space-time itself. And yet, as some astrophysicists conjecture, on "the other side" black holes are white holes emitting intense light.

The yogic work consists in spotting the beacon, drawing closer and closer to it, until we realize that the source of light beyond the *buddhi*'s Fresnel lens is our essential nature. In the moment of that realization, we *become* the source of light only to find that we are also the world beyond the light tower. We are the source of light, Fresnel lens, lighthouse, the cliff upon which the lighthouse stands, the vast ocean beyond it, and indeed all the visible and invisible realms of the unimaginably vast universe. Such is the glory of spiritual enlightenment. It surpasses the so-called enlightenment of rationalists like Descartes by astronomical magnitudes.

Guided by his trusted reason, Descartes arrived at a concept of God and the world that few today take seriously. For him, God was the great mechanic who fashioned the universe like a clock, wound it up, and now, satisfied with his handiwork, watches the world's progress through the ages. This deism makes no allowance for the mystical impulse in us. There is no spiritual poetry in Descartes' philosophy by which we could rise to the recognition of the Divine as our home. God is forever apart from his creatures.

By contrast, the key message of Vedanta is that there is no gulf between the Divine and the world; that to assume such a separation is a distortion of the truth, and is the root cause of our individual and collective experience of suffering (*duhkha*). On the contrary, the Vedanta philosophers and sages proclaim that our happiness lies in the discovery that there is no unbridgeable chasm between the Divine, or ultimate Reality, and us: The Divine is our true identity beyond all the many personae that we play out in daily life.

Jnana-yoga is virtually identical with Vedanta. This implies that, unlike Patanjali's Classical Yoga which is dualistic, *jnana-yoga* is based on the metaphysics of nondualism. According to most schools of this Hindu tradition, our perception of a universe rich in distinct forms and beings is a distortion of the truth. In reality, those multiple forms and beings are all appearances or forms of one and the same Being, called *brahman* or *atman*.

The term *jnana-yoga* is first mentioned in the *Bhagavad-Gita* (III.3), a pre-Christian work. Here the God-man Krishna declares that he has since time immemorial taught two ways of life—*jnana-yoga* for the *samkhyas* and *karma-yoga* ("Yoga of action") for the *yogins*. In this context, a *samkhya* is not so much an adherent of the Samkhya school of thought as a practitioner of wisdom, a traveler on the path of illumination, a *jnanin*.

Krishna equates *jnana-yoga* with *buddhi-yoga*. As we have seen, the *buddhi* is the faculty of wisdom, the higher mind in which the primary quality of *sattva* predominates. *Sattva* means literally "being-ness" or "real-ness." It is the principle of lucidity. It is present to one degree or another in all forms and beings. But it predominates in the *buddhi*, which is both a level of existence and an elevated mental function.

Every conceivable phenomenon, whether on the physical level or in other dimensions of cosmic existence, is the product of the interplay of the three primary forces of Nature (*prakriti*)—*sattva, rajas,* and *tamas*. The *buddhi* is deemed the very first and purest product

of the process of evolution by which forms and beings are manifested on various levels of existence.

All this is ancient wisdom. In a certain sense, the *Bhagavad-Gita*
merely articulates what had long been taught in esoteric circles by
word of mouth. In essence, *jnana-yoga* is present already in the
2800-year-old *Brihad-Aranyaka-Upanishad*. In this scripture, we
hear the utterances of great sages like Yajnavalkya and King Janaka,
who possess the secret wisdom of the Absolute (*brahman*). They
challenge the clever theologians and would-be mystics of their time
in dialogues that cost the loser his head, at least figuratively.

In this scripture we also encounter for the first time the teaching
of the two types of *brahman*, the lower and the higher. The lower
brahman is the world of form, and the higher *brahman* is the
formless Reality, which alone is immortal and blissful.

In the *Brihad-Aranyaka-Upanishad*, we also find the teaching of
neti neti ("not this, not that"), which is the bedrock of *jnana-yoga*.
Jnana-yoga can be characterized as a path of negation. It destroys
ignorance. It does not create new knowledge but merely removes
the obstruction to the truth that is always the same. The procedure
of *neti neti* was first communicated by the wise Yajnavalkya when
he instructed the brahmin Shakalya thus:

> That Self is not this, not that. It is intangible, for it cannot be grasped.
> It is incorruptible, for it cannot be corrupted. It is unattached, for it
> does not attach itself [to anything]. It is unbounded. It is not agitated.
> It is not injured. [6]

Yajnavalkya further described the nature of the transcendental
Self in a conversation with his spiritually inclined wife Maitreyi. He
remarked that after death there is no consciousness (*samjna*), which
confused Maitreyi greatly. Thereupon Yajnavalkya elucidated his
curious comment in the following classic passage:

> There is no consciousness after death] because [only] where there is
> apparent duality (*dvaita*), there one sees one another; there one
> smells one another; there one hears one another; there one speaks to
> one another; there one thinks of one another; there one understands
> one another. [But] where, verily, everything has become only the Self,
> then whereby and whom would one smell? Then whereby and whom
> would one see? Then whereby and whom would one hear? Then
> whereby and to whom would one speak? Then whereby and of

whom would one think? Then whereby and whom would one know? Whereby would one know him by whom one knows all this? Indeed, whereby would one know the Knower (*vijnatri*)? [7]

The Self is not conscious in the ordinary sense of the word. However, it is also not unconscious. It is, rather, pure awareness or superconsciousness (*cit*). All other attributes are simply super-impositions, projections of the mind. For the Self to reveal itself in its native splendor, all these projections must be withdrawn, or pierced through. This is achieved by means of the *via negativa* of the *neti neti* method.

This negative approach is succinctly illustrated in the *Nirvana-Shatka* ("Six [Stanzas] about Extinction"), which is one of the many didactic poems attributed to Shankara. The full text reads as follows:

I am not the mind or the wisdom faculty (*buddhi*), the I-sense, or thought; neither hearing nor the tongue; neither the nose nor the eyes; nor am I ether, earth, fire, and air. I am Shiva in the form of awareness (*cit*) and bliss (*ananda*). I am Shiva. (vs. 1)

I am not what is called the life-force (*prana*), nor am I the five airs [circulating in the body]; nor the seven [bodily] constituents; nor the five [bodily] sheaths. I am also not mouth, hands, feet, genitals, and anus. I am Shiva in the form of awareness and bliss. I am Shiva. (vs. 2)

I have neither hatred nor passion, neither greed nor delusion; neither exhilaration nor the mood of envy. I am without virtue or prosperity, without lust or liberation. I am Shiva in the form of awareness. I am Shiva. (vs. 3)

[In me there is] neither good nor evil, neither happiness nor suffering, neither *mantra* nor pilgrimage, neither the *Vedas* nor sacrifices. I am not food, the consumer, or [the process of] eating. I am Shiva in the form of awareness and bliss. I am Shiva. (vs. 4)

I am not [subject to] death, fear, or category of birth. I have no father and mother, [in fact, I have] no birth. I have no relatives and friends, no teacher and pupils. I am Shiva in the form of awareness and bliss. I am Shiva. (vs. 5)

I am undifferentiated, of formless form. Due to [my] omnipresence I am everywhere [present for the benefit of] all the senses. I am neither in bondage nor in liberation, immeasurable. I am Shiva in the form of awareness and bliss. I am Shiva. (vs. 6)

Here Shiva is not a specific deity of the Hindu pantheon but a symbol for the Absolute itself. The deities are all part of the relative dimension of existence. They belong to the "lower" *brahman*, also called *shabda-brahman* or the "voiced Absolute," that is, the Reality as it can be articulated in thought and speech. The Greeks called this the logos, a term corresponding to the Sanskrit *shabda*, which also means "word."

Ultimately, only the higher *brahman* is real. And it is this real *brahman* with which the sage wants to identify. To do so, he must learn to discriminate between what is real and unreal. This intuitive act of discrimination is known as *viveka*.

But there is another important ingredient of *jnana-yoga*, which is suggested in the story of Yajnavalkya. His instruction of Maitreyi coincided with an important turning-point in his life. For he announced to Maitreyi and Katyayani, his second wife, that he had decided to abandon his householder existence in favor of full renunciation (*samnyasa*). He was about to adopt the lifestyle of a *parama-hamsa* or "supreme swan"—a bird symbolizing self-sufficiency. Discrimination is one wing and renunciation is the other. Both are necessary for the "supreme swan's" flight to the Absolute.

In the fifteenth century the path of *jnana-yoga* was systematized by Sadananda in his *Vedanta-Sara* (15–25). We see from Sadananda's outline of the "limbs" of this Yoga of wisdom that discrimination and renunciation are its foundation:

1. *Viveka* or discrimination
2. *Viraga* or dispassion
3. *Shat-sampatti* ("six attainments"), *viz.*,
   a) *shama* or tranquillity
   b) *dama* or sense-restraint
   c) *uparati* or abstention from actions that are not relevant to the maintenance of bodily existence or the pursuit of enlightenment
   d) *titiksha* or endurance
   e) *samadhana* or mental collectedness
   f) *shraddha* or faith, which is not mere belief
4. *Mumukshutva* or impulse toward liberation

Shankara, in his commentary on the *Brahma-Sutra* (I.1.4), mentions the above limbs with the exception of mental collectedness. He adds *shravana* or "listening" to the sacred lore, *manana* or "pondering," and *nididhyasana* or "meditation." These are also defined in the *Vedanta-Sara* (182; 191–192). The same manual (200–208) even defines the eight "limbs" of Classical Yoga, presumably as an alternative to the above path. They are essentially the same.

Just as important as discrimination and renunciation is the impulse toward liberation (*mumukshutva*), without which there can be no Self-realization. Although Sadananda and other authorities of Vedanta explain *mumukshutva* as the "desire (*iccha*) for liberation," it is really not so much a desire as a reorientation of one's whole being toward the Divine. It is the will to receive the revelation of gnosis, or *jnana,* in which the narrow ego-sense is absent and the world and our body-mind glow as the all-comprising singular Reality.

NOTES

1. R. Descartes, *Discourse on Method* (La Salle, IL: Open Court, 1946), p. 17.

2. *A Practical Guide to Integral Yoga: Extracts Compiled from the Writings of Sri Aurobindo and The Mother* (Pondicherry, India: Sri Aurobindo Ashram, 1955), pp. 241–242.

3. P. Brunton, *The Notebooks of Paul Brunton,* vol. 1: *Perspectives: The Timeless Way of Wisdom* (Burdett, NY: Larson Publications, 1984), p. 263.

4. The Sanskrit word *buddhi* stems from the verbal root *budh,* meaning "to be awake."

5. The word *manas* is derived from the verbal root *man,* meaning "to think." This Sanskrit term is related to the Latin word *mens.*

6. *Brihad-Aranyaka-Upanishad* (III.9.26).

7. *Brihad-Aranyaka-Upanishad* (II.4.14).

7

THE WAY OF SELF-TRANSCENDING ACTION (KARMA-YOGA)

Of all the philosophical or spiritual questions that we could possibly ask ourselves, there are two *big* questions to which we must sooner or later find our own answers. The first question is *Why am I here?* This also comes in the form of *Who am I?* or *What does it all mean?* The second and closely related question, which is the focus of the present essay, is *What am I supposed to do with my life?* or *How should I live?*

Our secular Western culture provides us with a great variety of answers to these questions, which is one reason for the moral confusion we are witnessing. The other reason is the inadequacy of those answers, which portray human life as primarily a biological and social adventure, with nothing beyond that: The death of the cellular machine of the human body-mind is supposed to be the end of the story. And, from this point of view, it follows that it does not matter too much what we do with our lives and our planet.

The sacred traditions of the world offer us a different picture—a picture that is not only more compelling but also far more exciting. Thus, according to the Yoga tradition, we are essentially Consciousness-Energy (*cit-shakti*), and the physical body is merely an outer wrapping, a limited appearance of that Consciousness-Energy. There is so much more that is happening besides the familiar material processes. This picture opens up possibilities of experience for us that go far beyond the daily round of eating, drinking, sexing, working, playing, and socializing. The *yogin* discovers dimensions of experience that we barely suspect exist. Above all, however, the practitioner of Yoga assumes a different relationship to the ordinary activities of daily life; in fact, he or she transforms them. He or she makes the activities of daily life extraordinary occasions.

Not everyone is able to meditate profoundly, regularly, and consistently. Everyone is, however, able to practice what in India is known as *karma-yoga,* meaning literally "action Yoga." This Yoga consists in the sacred work of transforming one's everyday activities. It was first taught by the God-man Krishna, the enlightened teacher of prince Arjuna, on the eve of the greatest battle fought on ancient Indian soil. Krishna's teaching has been preserved in the *Bhagavad-Gita* ("Lord's Song"), the most famous Yoga scripture. In the third chapter of this "Song of the Lord," Krishna instructs Arjuna—and us—in what is called "skillful action."

Krishna argues that activity is an inseparable attribute of finite existence. Nothing that exists in the realm of Nature is, in the last analysis, inactive. Nature (*prakriti*), which is composed of three types of primary qualities (*guna*), is a perpetual motion machine. If it ceased to move even for a moment, the cosmos would collapse. This view coincides with the findings of modern physics, which has revealed to us a universe that is continually vibrating.

Therefore, concludes Krishna, it does not make much sense to want to abstain from action. Mere inactivity is not the answer to our existential problems. It is fine to renounce the world and dedicate one's life to contemplating the Divine, providing one can really do it. But few people have the necessary stamina for the rigors of such a solitary lifestyle. Besides, argues Krishna, there is a better way to Self-realization (or God-realization) than renunciation. And that is to continue to be active *but* to act free from egoic attachment. In this way, the continuation of human life is ensured, while at the same time it is being transformed by one's self-transcending disposition.

Krishna's activist gospel, then, does not ask us to carry on as usual. True, the *karma-yogin* or the *karma-yogini* continues to get up in the morning, eat breakfast, go to work, interact with people during the day, return home, eat dinner, spend time with the family, read, listen to music, make love, and sleep. *But* he or she endeavors, by degrees, to do all this with a subtle yet significant difference: All of these actions are engaged in the spirit of self-surrender. In other words, they are all opportunities to go beyond mere egoic preferences and fixations and to cultivate instead quiet awareness and communion with the Divine.

An important aspect of the practice of *karma-yoga* is the non-neurotic disinterest in what Krishna calls the "fruit" of one's actions. Ordinarily, our actions are governed by so-called ulterior motives—those mostly hidden expectations that would see us rewarded for our deeds. For instance, by putting in an extra hour at work, we secretly, or otherwise, hope to impress the boss. By taking our children to sporting events on Saturdays, we hope for them to share our own excitement, or by sending them to medical school, we seek to live out our own dreams in their lives.

By helping an elderly or blind person cross the street, we expect, below the threshold of our conscious mind, to be thanked and thus receive an emotional boost. Or, more subtly, we may do things out of a sense of duty, but without heart. In that case, our actions remain as self-involved as ever. Grim determination is not a substitute for the spirit of self-transcendence.

Evidently *karma-yoga* requires a healthy dose of self-knowledge, because in order to engage activities on the basis of self-transcendence rather than self-interest or even self-indulgence, we must first know how that self presents itself in our own case. We must know the patterns of our own egoic personality. Fortunately, we do not have to postpone our practice of *karma-yoga* until we have thoroughly understood ourselves. We can start paying attention—right now—to the hidden motives in our activities, and self-knowledge will grow step by step, as will our capacity to transcend those egoic motives.

Krishna adds another important point to this whole consideration. He argues that we must not only act without egoic attachment, but we must also choose to do the *right* kind of action. For Krishna, who lived well over two thousand years ago, this meant essentially to act in accordance with the social and spiritual wisdom of his day. It would be foolhardy to try to transplant that wisdom to our far more complex contemporary situation, though we can of course learn from it.

We must find out for ourselves what is right and what is wrong in each case. For instance, while it is completely appropriate for a practitioner of *karma-yoga* to earn a living, it may not be appropriate for him or her to work in an ammunitions factory or a slaughterhouse, or in a stressful environment. This is where one must exercise discrimination.

At any rate, for the *karma-yogin* or *karma-yogini*, work is not merely a means of economic survival or psychic gratification; it is primarily service (*seva*). And this, in a way, is true of all his or her actions, whether in the workplace or at home. What the practitioner of *karma-yoga* is serving is the physical, mental, and spiritual welfare of others, including nonhuman beings. The *Bhagavad-Gita* speaks of this as the ideal of *loka-samgraha*, which literally means "world gathering," or the bringing together of the world, that is, the protection and nurturing of all beings on this planet and anywhere else.

"Mahatma" Gandhi embodied this ideal to perfection, and it is not surprising that we learn from his autobiography that early in his life he had imbibed the spirit of the *Gita*, which he tried to memorize. In his own words:

> . . . to me the *Gita* became an infallible guide of conduct. It became my dictionary of daily reference. Just as I turned to the English dictionary for the meanings of English words that I did not understand, I turned to this dictionary of conduct for a ready solution of all my troubles and trials. Words like *aparigraha* (non-possession) and *samabhava* (equability) gripped me . . . I understood the *Gita* teaching of non-possession to mean that those who desired salvation should act like the trustee who, though having control over great possessions, regards not an iota of them as his own.[1]

Upon closer examination it will be found that skillful action—that is, right action performed without egoic attachment—is inherently loving. When we dethrone the ego, which thinks of itself as the "owner" of objects, beings, ideas, and experiences, we also cease to exert our will over them. Instead, we are more likely to treat others, including apparently inanimate things, with reverence. We see the greater Life manifesting in everything.

This "vision of sameness" (*sama-darshana*) is the foundation for the crucially important attitude of nonharming (*ahimsa*), which Gandhi exemplified in his personal and political life. As he put it:

> To see the universal and all-pervading Spirit of Truth face to face one must be able to love the meanest of creation as oneself. And a man who aspires after that cannot afford to keep out of any field of life. That

is why my devotion to Truth has drawn me into the field of politics; and I can say without the slightest hesitation, and yet in all humility, that those who say that religion has nothing to do with politics do not know what religion means.[2]

Gandhi continued:

Identification with everything that lives is impossible without self-purification; without self-purification the observance of the law of Ahimsa must remain an empty dream; God can never be realized by one who is not pure of heart.[3]

Self-transcending action thus presupposes both love (*bhakti*) and discernment (*jnana*) between what is real and unreal. This makes *karma-yoga* ultimately as demanding a way to Self-realization as any other spiritual orientation. However, it seems particularly suited to the active Western disposition, and therefore it is, of all the Yogas, the most accessible starting-point for anyone seriously interested in applying the ancient Yoga wisdom in daily life.

If we apply ourselves to the principles of *karma-yoga,* we may well find, as Sri Aurobindo noted, that our actions remain outwardly the same.[4] The real work we are challenged to undertake concerns our inner life. Yet, our new inner disposition will inevitably shine through our actions as well. We may still perform the same steps in washing dishes, for instance, but our movements and comportment will be calm and balanced.

In fact, we should fully expect a subtle but significant difference in anyone who has genuinely been inwardly reborn. That difference is a matter of the Spirit's or Self's luster irradiating, to whatever degree, his or her body-mind and actions. When this is the case, life is lived in simplicity and with a quiet strength. We become transparent to ourselves and to others, and our inner radiance spontaneously kindles the spiritual flame in others.

NOTES

1. M.K. Gandhi, *An Autobiography: The Story of My Experiments with Truth* (Boston, MA: Beacon Press, 1957), p. 265.

2. *Ibid.*, p. 504.

3. *Ibid.*, p. 504.

4. See R.A. McDermott, ed., *The Essential Aurobindo* (New York: Schocken Books, 1973), p. 116.

8

"WORSHIP ME WITH LOVE"—BHAKTI-YOGA

"All there is is love . . ." The Beatles and the flower children of the 1960s knew it: Love is what this world is all about. Not the world of competitiveness, apartheid, social problems, espionage, sabotage, economic progress, and war, but the world *in essence*. We have to step out of our daily skins to appreciate this fact, as did, to some extent, the dropouts of twenty or thirty years ago.

Of course, they were incurable romantics, reacting to the buttoned-down mentality of the older generation. But it is regrettable that their troubadour days are over, because our era is in need of the message of love, even simple talk or reminders about love. I do not mean sophomoric crushes, gushy emotionalism, syrupy neighborliness, or even the New Age kind of romantic, idealistic love between soul mates. Rather, what we need is love as an expression of the greater Reality in which we all inhere and where we are all truly united, since all distinctions are obsolete in it.

When we relax our habitual image of ourselves as egos wrapped in flesh, when we cut through our primal fear (*bhaya*), we get in touch with the power of love. Vedanta tells us that our essential nature is bliss (*ananda*) or happiness, which is another word for love. But love suggests a more active involvement than does bliss or happiness. Perhaps it would not be wrong to say that love is the *practice* of happiness.

In the Hindu tradition of *bhakti-yoga*, such love is variously called *bhakti* or *preman*. This love comes not from the mouth or the head. It is a matter of the heart, which epitomizes the entire bodily being. Love wells up from the *anahata-cakra*, the heart center, where the *yogin* perceives the "unstruck" (*anahata*) sound, the boom of eternity. [1]

Love, or bliss, is a radiant force that bubbles up in us and, in its characteristic superabundance, flows out from us. When we are in love with a person, our love spills over to everybody and everything; it is not confined to our beloved. We embrace all, and our loving embrace is infectious. Love is ecstatic, and it engenders love.

There is a great lesson in this, but a lesson that we seldom really learn, because as soon as we fall out of love with our beloved, we fall out of love with everyone and everything, including ourselves. Life looks drab again, or at least no longer quite as extraordinary, whereas our love or abundant happiness infused it with a vibrant vitality that made it enormously attractive.

Few people in our society know such love. It requires a great depth of feeling, and feeling is largely outlawed in our heady, patriarchal world. Feeling is different from emotionality. It is almost an extended form of the sense of touch. By comparison, emotions are mere local disturbances of the bodily field—anger, sorrow, fear, grief, excitement, envy, jealousy, or lust, even such apparently positive emotions as pleasure, self-satisfaction, or warm regard. Feeling transcends them all, just as it transcends our self-sense and our bodily image. In feeling, we reach out beyond the apparent walls of our body-mind.

Feeling—free feeling—is the carrier for the power of love. *Bhakti-yoga* is thus the discipline of self-transcending feeling-participation in the world at large. Significantly, the Sanskrit word *bhakti* comes from the verbal root *bhaj*, meaning "to participate in." Through and in love, we participate in the larger Life, in what the teachers of *bhakti-yoga* call the Divine Person. That transcendental Person, or *purusha-uttama,* is the universal soil from which springs all life.

Perhaps the flower children intuited something of this. But their "Yoga" was an unconscious one. It lacked self-knowledge, discipline, and the renunciation of what clear insight has revealed to be unreal or false about oneself. There can be no Yoga, no spiritual life, without self-understanding, disciplined self-application, and renunciation. So, *bhakti-yoga* contains elements of *jnana-yoga* (the Yoga of discriminative wisdom), *karma-yoga* (the Yoga of self-transcending action), and *samnyasa-yoga* (the Yoga of renunciation).

At the beginning of his *Bhakti-Sutra* ("Aphorisms on Love"), the legendary Sage Narada noted that *bhakti* is not a form of lust because it entails the spirit of renunciation (*nirodha*).[2] He explained renunciation as the consecration of all one's activities, whether religious or secular, to the Divine Person. Through this act of offering up one's works, a state of unification with the Divine is achieved.

This single-minded self-dedication is best epitomized in the spiritual passion of the shepherdesses for the God-man Krishna. According to legend, the shepherdesses (*gopi*), some of whom were married, were filled with a great longing whenever Krishna would play his flute.[3] Like the Pied Piper he beguiled and distracted them from their daily chores, irresistibly drawing them to him. When they had completely fallen in love with him, their hearts would be with the God-man even in his absence.

The story of Radha, Krishna's favorite shepherdess, relates how she pined for him like a love-sick girl. He would fuel her passion by prolonged periods of absence. The story is a wonderful allegory of the play between the psyche and the higher Reality, which reveals itself in all its glory now and again, leaving us with a growing desire for divine union. The love mystics of medieval Christendom, notably Saint Bernard of Clairvaux, Saint Theresa of Avila, and Saint John of the Cross, have bequeathed to us dramatic accounts of that miraculous work in the depth of the human psyche.[4]

Love, then, is not merely a temporary high, a feeling of elation. It must be cultivated as a continuous spiritual disposition. We must love even when we feel slighted, hurt, angered, bored, or depressed —especially in those moments. *Bhakti-yoga* is the steady application of our feeling capacity in all life situations. Even in our worst moments, we must extend our love, or fundamental respect, to all others. Even though life consists of peaks and valleys, our overall commitment must be to what is revealed in our brief spells on the peaks.

We are not expected to always walk around "happy"—at least not while we are unenlightened. In fact, even enlightened beings experience emotional ups and downs, but there is an underlying current of bliss that is always accessible to them, or even continuously present for them, regardless of their momentary states, which may include annoyance, anger, grief, as is clear from the classical descriptions as well as contemporary accounts.

Traditionally, *bhakti-yoga* harnesses a person's feeling-energy so that all his or her impulses get directed toward the Divine. For many of us, who have been brought up in a blatantly secular culture, this is difficult to understand and to do. We may find it easier to love concrete beings than what is likely to be a merely abstract God. Also, in the past, other beings have often been ignored and ill-treated in the name of a false devotion to the Divine. We cannot reach the Divine over the maimed bodies, persecuted minds, or broken hearts of our fellow beings. Striving for enlightenment or God-realization must also not be an exclusive, selfish undertaking. The practice of love must be universal. We are obliged to love—not blindly but most profoundly.

There is, however, a certain danger in focusing our love on other conditional beings, and that is that we may confuse spirituality and love with "doing good," or exercising a merely social morality. If our loving of others is to be true, we must see in them, and respond to, that which is real and eternal, bright and blissful. As Sage Yajna-valkya instructed his students more than two thousand years ago: We do not love another for the sake of their wealth, personality, or beauty—but for the sake of the transcendental Self (*atman*), which is the same in all of us.

What does the practice of *bhakti* involve? First of all, it most certainly does not mean that we should love others *abstractly*. Love is not merely a wonderful feeling we have about others. It is not merely a benign or kind thought. We have every right to distrust a person who continually assures us of his or her love, but typically fails to express or manifest it to us and to others. To distrust someone, however, does not mean to reject him or her, or to be otherwise unloving ourselves.

Love is demonstrated in action. But more than being demonstrated in action, love *is* action. We can sit in our room for an entire lifetime and think loving thoughts about other people, but if we never express our love to them, if we never actively share our love with them, we will not have loved.

Mother Teresa of Calcutta is someone in whom the spirit of *bhakti-yoga* is very much alive. Every day of her life, she actively shares her love with men, women, and children who are spurned by the larger society. Of course, we need not travel to Calcutta or treat lepers; yet, if we want to be *bhaktas*, or practitioners of love, we must certainly imbibe something of the spirit in which she conducts her life.

The fact is that we are not incapable of love but are only afraid to love. Our great fear is that we will not be loved in return, or that we will be outright rejected. There is of course no guarantee that our self-giving in love will evoke love in others, although love *is* infectious.

For our love not to crumble under the onslaught of the lovelessness around us, it must be a surplus in us, and it must be a steady force in our lives. Who can deny the lovelessness that surrounds us? It shows itself in a thoughtless remark, an inappropriate silence, a tasteless joke, an aggressive move, turning away from another's pain, the failure to really listen, the pursuit of orgasm at the expense of caring—all the many ways in which we unconsciously hurt one another, out of ignorance, inattention, or sheer unwillingness to make a relational gesture.

We must try to understand the robotic ways in which we block out love. We must become sensitive to our own habitual lovelessness, so that love can become an attractive force in our lives. If you imagine that you already love, examine your life more thoroughly. It is quite revealing how little we in fact love when we start paying attention to our actions and relationships. But unless we are realistic about our lack of love, we can never go beyond our present state.

We must love *concretely*, that is to say, we must give our love to *specific* beings. And we might as well start at home, with our wife or husband and our children, and not least our parents. What we will find is that sometimes loving them is easy, and at other times it is the hardest thing imaginable.

To really love is a great discipline, because we must love stably and consistently and regardless of whether or not our love is returned. In other words, we must love despite our likes and dislikes—that is, despite our selves or egos. We must simply *allow* love to be a transformative force in our lives. *Allowing* is the key. And this is not a passive but an active discipline. It is the discipline of *bhakti-yoga.*

If we truly love, we discover that our love is concrete but not *confined* to specific beings. We must not confuse spiritual love with the feelings of affinity, friendship, or sexual attraction, or with being nice. Real love knows no content and boundaries. In a way, it is true to say that we are able either to love everyone or no one. *Bhakti* is all-inclusive. It shines through us and on to others without qualification. Its real "object" is the Divine itself, which is also its source. Love is thus unconditional. It is an intimate embrace of all beings and things in their entirety. As psychologist John Welwood commented:

> Whenever our heart opens to another person, we experience a moment of unconditional love. People commonly imagine that unconditional love is a high or distant ideal, one that is difficult, if not impossible, to realize. Yet though it may be hard to put into everyday practice, its nature is quite simple and ordinary: opening and responding to another person's being without reservation.[5]

Love is not something we can "do." To say that we "make" love is a contradiction in terms. We only "make" our bodies mingle and our nervous systems tingle. But love is either the case, or it is not. It is a state of being that is either true or not true of us. If it is true of us, we cannot help but love all and everyone, regardless of whether or not they offer us gratitude, friendship, or sexual fulfillment.

Genuine love asks for nothing in return, though it always works toward duplicating itself in others. Thus, the greatest reward for a person who practices the discipline of love is that another being has become illumined by that love and is now carrying the gift to others.

I said earlier that love has little to do with being nice. In fact, love is being present as a radiant force that comes from beyond the lesser self and reaches out toward that which is beyond the lesser self of others. When that radiance is true of us, we may feel moved to take actions that, by ordinary standards, are not particularly nice. As the French essayist Michel Eyquem Montaigne put it: "He loves little who loves by rule." This is an echo of Saint Augustine who said: "Love and do what thou wilt."

To be present as love does not, for instance, preclude the possibility of our feeling angry with someone, though in our anger we do not seek to obliterate the other, take revenge, or otherwise seek to further ourselves. Christians will remember the New Testament story of Jesus' stern handling of the money lenders in the temple of Jerusalem.

Buddhists are well acquainted with the story of the famous Tibetan teacher Marpa who was known for his fierce anger as well as his enlightenment. These two facts appear irreconcilable, unless one knows that Marpa's fierceness was for the sake of his disciples' enlightenment. He treated Milarepa and the other students so harshly only because he loved them and wanted to guide them to their own discovery of the ultimate Reality. Today, Milarepa is cele–brated as Tibet's greatest *yogin*.

The love of the teacher for the student is a special form of the love the enlightened adept feels for all beings. When the disciple has awakened to the same intensity of love, the teacher has accomplished his or her task. But whether or not our spiritual practice is guided by a living master, we are always facing the same "impossible" demand: to be present *as* love in all circumstances.

For a long time, all we will see is our failure to meet this demand. But this need not discourage us, because in every moment we have a new opportunity to practice that love. We must become fools who are willing to risk again and again that simple response of embracing the Divine in the form of specific beings and things.

NOTES

1. The *anahata-cakra*, which is also known as the *hrit-padma* ("heart lotus"), is one of seven principal psychoenergetic centers of the body.

2. See the translation by Swami Tyagisananda, *Narada Bhakti Sutras* (Mylapore, India: Ramakrishna Math, 5th ed. 1972). For further study, see the following works: Bhaktivedanta Swami, *The Nectar of Devotion* (New York: Bhaktivedanta Book Trust, 1979); Swami Sivananda, *Essence of Bhakti Yoga* (Sivanandanagar, India: Sivananda Literature Research Institute, 1960); Swami Vivekananda, *Bhakti-Yoga* (Calcutta: Advaita Ashram, 1970).

3. For the playful relationship between Krishna and the shepherdess, see D.R. Kinsley, *The Divine Player: A Study of Krsna Lila* (Delhi: Banarsidass, 1979).

4. See G. Feuerstein, *Sacred Sexuality* (Los Angeles: J.P. Tarcher, 1992).

5. J. Welwood, *Journey of the Heart: Intimate Relationship and the Path of Love* (New York: HarperCollins, 1990), p. 39.

9

THE KRIYA-YOGA OF PATANJALI

Yoga is a kind of technology or, if you prefer, counter-technology. It is the technology of consciousness transformation. This is, of course, true of all forms of genuine Yoga. But not every school or branch of the proliferative tradition of Yoga has such an elaborate theoretical underpinning as Patanjali's Classical Yoga.

For this reason, Patanjali's *Yoga-Sutra* holds special significance for students of Yoga. This Sanskrit work, which is as old as the Christian gospels, defines important yogic concepts. Naturally, within the compass of this short tract, consisting of a mere 195 aphorisms (*sutra*), one must not expect a complete exposition of the doctrinal structure of Classical Yoga. This was not Patanjali's purpose. His aphorisms were simply intended to aid the memory of initiates of Classical Yoga. Many things were not even mentioned, as is clear when we read the early commentaries on the *Yoga-Sutra,* which fill some of the gaps. Modern students of the *Yoga-Sutra* therefore have to be patient and diligent.

Patanjali's school is generally referred to as *the* "Yoga system" (*yoga-darshana*). It is also widely known as the "eight-limbed Yoga" (*ashta-anga-yoga*). However, as I have tried to show in various books, the section in the *Yoga-Sutra* dealing with the eight "limbs" (*anga*) of the yogic path is very likely a quote from a previously existing *Sutra*. Patanjali's own teaching is more appropriately called *kriya-yoga.* This expression is found in aphorism II.1, which reads: "Asceticism, study, and devotion to the Lord [constitute] the Yoga of [ritual] action" (*tapah svadhyaya-ishvara-pranidhanani kriya-yogah*). Asceticism (*tapas*), study (*svadhyaya*), and devotion to the Lord (*ishvara-pranidhana*) are the three principal means of Patanjali's Yoga. They are sacred acts (*kriya*).

They fall under the category of "practice" (*abhyasa*). The complementary category is "dispassion" (*vairagya*). Together, practice and dispassion provide the dynamic of spiritual life, as understood by Patanjali. The eight limbs are moral restraint (*yama*), self-restraint (*niyama*), posture (*asana*), breath control (*pranayama*), sensory inhibition (*pratyahara*), concentration (*dharana*), meditation (*dhyana*), and ecstasy (*samadhi*). These can be considered as subcategories of asceticism, though study and devotion to the Lord also appear under self-restraint. For Patanjali, at any rate, they held special importance.

The objective of *kriya-yoga*, as we learn from aphorism II.2, is the cultivation of ecstasy and the attenuation of the "causes-of-suffering" (*klesha*). The ulterior motive for this psychotechnology is, according to aphorism II.16, the prevention of future suffering (*duhkha*). For Patanjali, as for Gautama the Buddha, the source of all suffering is spiritual ignorance (*avidya*). This is in fact the primary *klesha*. From it spring the I-sense (*asmita*), attachment (*raga*), aversion (*dvesha*), and the "will-to-live" (*abhinivesha*). Patanjali explains these five *kleshas* as follows (II.5-II.9):

Ignorance is seeing [that which is] eternal, pure, joyful, and the Self in [that which is] ephemeral, impure, sorrowful, and the nonself (*anatman*).

"I-am-ness" (*asmita*) is the identification as it were of the powers of vision [i.e., the mind] and "vision-er" [i.e., the Self].

Attachment is [that which] rests on pleasant [experiences].

Aversion is [that which] rests on sorrowful [experiences].

The "will-to-live," flowing along [by its] own momentum, is rooted thus even in the sages.

These five "causes-of-suffering" furnish the dynamic of ordinary life. They are the motivational matrix of the unenlightened psyche. *Kriya-yoga* seeks to undermine this innate pattern so that the person can recover his or her authentic being, which is the Self. Self-realization is the only means of disrupting the cycle of repeated births and deaths to which the unenlightened being is subject.

The five *kleshas* urge the individual to feel, think, will, and act. These functions leave either positive or negative traces in the depths of the human psyche from where they instigate new activities and experiences that, in turn, generate further traces. This psychological model is central to *kriya-yoga*. Long before modern psychology, Patanjali invented the significant concept of the "depth-mind," which he called *smriti* (literally "memory"). It is in this depth-mind that the psychic residue of one's actions and experiences is stored.

Like most other yogic concepts, the notion of the depth-mind is not merely a speculative construct. *Yogins* do not tend to indulge in philosophical flights, but their theorizing always has a definite and concrete purpose. Thus, the idea of the depth-mind is meant to explain and facilitate a very important aspect of the yogic process. The depth-mind can be understood as the total configuration of a person's psychic residue from past volitional activity.

Any action, whether deliberate or involuntary, creates a corresponding disposition in the deepest recesses of the mind. These dispositions combine, presumably on the basis of association by similarity, to form complex chains and concatenations rather like crisscross tracks in the sand or snow. Of course, this three-dimensional imagery is not entirely appropriate because we are dealing here with immaterial realities rather than substances with spatial extension.

These configurations would be of no practical consequence if they were not the driving factors behind all our future volitional activity. Thus the depth-mind is not simply a bottomless ditch into which the content of our self-expression is dumped. But it is a "radioactive" force, the nurturing ground that engenders new impulses toward self-expression.

This dynamic aspect of the depth-mind is captured in the Sanskrit term *samskara*, which means literally "activator." Each unit of experience, or self-expression, creates a *samskara* in the depth-mind. Patanjali does not tell us exactly how the subliminal activators determine our mental activity. He simply asserts that they do. His claim can be verified very easily.

Try to sit completely still, silencing your thoughts and internal images. How many seconds are you able to do this exercise before thoughts and images intervene again? Even if you should succeed to curb your mind for ten seconds, with practice you would find that beneath the apparent stillness is a constant rumble of sensations and feelings. The depth-mind is constantly at work.

Before we know it, we are witnessing verbal fragments, images, thoughts, and sudden emotions bubbling up from below the surface of the mind: serious and funny ideas, blurred images and vivid panoramic flashbacks, feelings of guilt, shame, anger, or fear. We discover how very difficult it is merely to observe and not get involved in the drama that is being enacted on the stage of our inner theater. As we watch the play we tend to become gradually and imperceptibly more involved until we have completely lost our original stance of a detached witness. All of a sudden, we identify with the drama.

The mind is a billowy sea with numerous whirlpools in which we continually lose our true identity as the Self. It is by force of habit that we cannot remain observers for very long. And "habit" is merely another word for the *samskara* chains that form the lattice of the depth-mind. Patanjali employs the term *vasana* ("trait") for these subliminal configurations composed of similar *samskaras*. He also refers to them collectively as "karmic deposit" (*karma-ashaya*).

Patanjali's model reminds one of certain modern theories of learning, conditioning, and habit formation. However, there is one all-important difference between these contemporary theories and Patanjali's formulations. According to Patanjali, only a very small segment of the total network of subliminal traits is the product of the present life's mental activity. The larger part of the depth-mind was in existence before our present birth and was indeed instrumental to our assumption of a new body. The depth-mind is the crystallization of a person's untold past existences, and it is the medium that regulates the entire process of re-embodiment. The doctrine of re-incarnation, or *punar-janman,* is one of the fundamental axioms of Yoga philosophy.

The practical implications of this belief are enormous. On one side, it is intended to account for the fact that people are endowed with different mental capacities and that their lives proceed along idiosyncratic lines that cannot be satisfactorily explained in terms of environmental or other external factors. On the other side, far from relieving a person from all responsibility, the teaching of reincarnation constitutes a challenge to actively determine his or her future lot. Nothing would be more wrong and destructive than to regard the doctrine of repeated births as a convenient excuse for a fatalistic attitude. Rather it should be seen as urging us to accept our individual "starting point," however disadvantageous it may seem, as the direct outcome of our previous mental activities, and to make the best of our life within the given parameters.

Although the "gravity pull" of the subliminal deposits is exceedingly powerful—"old habits die hard"—the yogic adepts assure us that we can overcome it through conscious work on ourselves. In fact, Patanjali insists that we can completely transcend the forces of destiny, and this optimistic assumption underlies all forms of Yoga. We can outwit karma by assuming the position of the witnessing Self, by disidentifying with the body-mind that *is* the karmic fruit of previous lives and of present volitional activities.

As a product of Nature (*prakriti*), the body-mind—which includes individuated consciousness (*citta*)—has no awareness of its own. It is rather like a clock that ticks until the wound-up spring is unwound. This mechanical imagery is not at all inappropriate here. The dualist metaphysics of Classical Yoga corresponds to the materialist view proposed in the eighteenth century by Descartes, who regarded the body as a machine. So long as we identify with the body-mind, we are also subject to its laws. However, the moment we identify with the Self, the principle of awareness (*cit*), we become disentangled from the fate of the body-mind.

Although Patanjali does not discuss the philosophical issue of free will in his *Yoga-Sutra*, his yogic technology implies that we can determine our future. We can choose to live either as the body-mind or as the Self. Different destinies follow from this choice. Already in the pre-Christian *Bhagavad-Gita* (XVI.6), the God-man Krishna speaks of "divine" (*daiva*) and "demonic" (*asura*) destinies, which depend on whether we place our attention on spiritual matters or on earthly concerns. In aphorism IV.7, Patanjali distinguishes between the "black," the "white," and the "mixed" karma of ordinary mortals, and the karma of *yogins*, which is neither black nor white nor mixed because it tends toward Self-realization and thus toward the end of all future suffering in repeated births and deaths.

But the exercise of free will in the direction of Self-realization must not remain a mere good intention: It must be expressed in a definite course of action. This action (*kriya*) must countermand the production of subliminal activators and delimit their sphere of influence. Patanjali recognizes different stages in this process of control over the incessantly active depth-mind. According to aphorism II.4, the "causes-of-suffering" can be fully operative (*udara*), dormant (*prasupta*), intercepted (*vicchinna*), or attenuated (*tanu*). The *yogin*'s goal is the attenuation and, finally, the utter cessation of their functioning.

It is to this end that the practitioner of Yoga employs the various yogic "limbs," notably the practice of ecstasy. It is in its use of techniques of ecstatic self-transcendence that Yoga differs most profoundly from psychoanalysis, which also works with the depth-mind. Psychoanalysts assume that the depth-mind, the so-called unconscious, can be positively influenced and moderately controlled by means of intellectual insight into the causes of unconscious automaticities (neuroses, psychoses, etc.). The masters of Yoga, however, have long understood that insight is necessary but not sufficient to transcend the powers of the "unconscious."

Even insight produces subliminal activators, which fuel the depth-mind. The *yogin* is not satisfied with generating better *samskaras*. He wants to generate none at all and, more than that, dissolve the rest. According to Patanjali, this is possible only in the fire of ecstatic transcendence in *asamprajnata-samadhi*. This "supraconscious" ecstasy does not involve the powerful ego-habit and therefore generates a counter-*samskara* based on enlightenment, which slowly dissolves all the other *samskaras*. In other words, as we make a habit of Self-identification by regularly ascending into supraconscious ecstasy, we weaken the habit of self-identification, or ego-consciousness, when we return to the ordinary state of mind. In the end, the ordinary consciousness is what is extraordinary, because the advanced practitioner identifies less and less with the body-mind, until he permanently abides as the Self.

The "limbs" of Yoga are aids in this progressive shift away from the egoic identity. Yet, in the final analysis, the "causes-of-suffering" are overcome not through any specific exercise but solely by the act of disidentifying with the body-mind. As Patanjali states in aphorism II.17:

> The correlation between the "seer" [i.e., the Self] and the "seen"
> [i.e., the body-mind] is the cause [of that which is] to be overcome
> [i.e., future suffering].

The "correlation" (*samyoga*) between the body-mind and the transcendental Self, which is pure awareness, is beginningless. But it can be terminated. Yoga is in fact a graduated process of severing that connection through gnosis (*vidya*), through awakening as the Self beyond spiritual ignorance and suffering. Such Self-realization is liberation, freedom, or what Patanjali calls "aloneness" (*kaivalya*). The Self is "alone" (*kevala*) not because it is a windowless monad but because it transcends the mechanics of material Nature, whether visible or invisible. It is unaffected by karma, the law of action and reaction. It is merely witnessing the events unfolding in the cosmos.

As King Bhoja, a tenth-century commentator on the *Yoga-Sutra*, rightly noted, *yoga* is not so much "union" (*samyoga*) as "separation" (*viyoga*). It entails a process of sifting out the nonself from the Self, the unreal from the Real. The Real is the transcendental Self (*purusha*), which shines forth in its solitary splendor when we have successfully overcome our illusions about reality.

However, we must not think of the solitary Self as being lonely. Emotions belong to the body-mind, not the Self. Yet, in aphorism II.5, Patanjali indirectly describes the Self as being joyful (*sukha*). This corresponds to the description of the Self as pure bliss (*ananda*) in the tradition of Vedanta. But the Self's delight is not an emotional condition. Rather, like the Self's eternal nature or its power of awareness, that delight is an inalienable quality of Reality.

10

FAITH AND SURRENDER: A NEW LOOK AT THE EIGHTFOLD PATH OF YOGA

The eight "limbs" (*anga*) of Yoga have, rightly or wrongly, come to stand for the Yoga taught by Patanjali in his *Yoga-Sutra*. Generally, they are conceived as a series of stages that the spiritual practitioner ascends, rather like a staircase, to the ideal of liberation or Self-realization. This popular "vertical" interpretation of the eight limbs is not entirely convincing; for, clearly, some of them are to be practiced simultaneously. But the underlying idea of these limbs as a kind of organic whole is unchallengeable.

What is rarely considered, though, is the question of what exactly links together all these limbs to give one the impression of such unity. To say that they are all essential parts of the yogic enterprise would only be the obvious answer. What do they all have in common at the deepest level so that we can recognize them to be integral components of Yoga?

I would like to propose that this "missing link" is the practice of *surrender* and *faith*, which have nothing to do with quasi-religious emotionalism but, rather, are profound attitudes without which spiritual growth cannot occur. Before I go on to illustrate this point with regard to each constituent practice of the eightfold path, let me further explain what I mean by these two terms.

Linguistically, the word "surrender" is composed of the prefix *sur-* and the verb *render*, meaning "to deliver over, to yield up, to render unto." The word is used in a variety of ways: to relinquish an office or entitlement, to offer up for sale an insurance policy, to capitulate to the enemy, to give oneself up to the authorities, or to succumb to despair. In each case the act involved is one of making over, or handing over, something.

In Yoga, as in all other forms of spirituality, this surrender consists not so much in any external transaction but primarily in an inner attitude or response. This attitude is one of "standing back" from oneself, a deliberate relaxation of the boundaries of the ego. What this involves is best indicated by the act of emotional and physical surrender between lovers—a further important usage of the word. In fact, when I once spoke on this subject to a group of Yoga enthusiasts, this was their first and foremost association.

Nor was the group's association of surrender with the act of yielding between lovers entirely positive. There was a feeling that such sexual-emotional surrender is usually a unilateral affair, that it is expected of the woman but that it does not match the masculine "aggressive" self-image of the male lover. Undoubtedly, women have widely been and still are exploited sexually, and an ideology of surrender would fit the bill of the male chauvinists perfectly. However, the present consideration does not focus on these social patterns.

Here we are interested in the dynamics of a *true* loving relationship between sexual partners. They are by definition "equal," for their surrender must be mutual. Of course, such mutual surrender presupposes great individual maturity. Starry-eyed teenagers who have "fallen" in love are incapable of this act, although they may seem to outsiders, and to themselves, to be completely absorbed in one another; in fact, their "love" is a subconscious projection of themselves onto the partner. Strictly speaking, they love themselves in the other. Hence, when reality hits, they "fall out of" love again. That not only teenagers but also so-called adults are victims to this "falling in and out of" love is a commentary on their level of maturity.

I am making so much of this because in *spiritual* surrender, the element of mature love is present as well. When the lover surrenders "body and soul" to the beloved, really what she (or more rarely, he) yields up is the usual self-identification with the body and with bodily and emotional and even mental processes. There is a melting away of conventional propriety, shame, and guilt. Indeed, lovers delight in pouring their hearts out to one another, in confiding long-kept secrets or long-cherished hopes, and in "daring" each other to demonstrate their love by overcoming inhibitions and taboos.

They are self-forgetful—or so it seems. At least they are on the way to being self-forgetful. That they never quite succeed is as obvious as it is subtle. Their surrender is necessarily incomplete, because their love is imperfect. This lies in the nature of ordinary human love, however extraordinary it may be by conventional standards.

Perfect love is possible only with regard to a perfect "object" or, to be more precise, when love is without a specific object but includes all possible objects, the whole universe. This, again, means that perfect love is possible only when there is no ego to create the usual barrier—however tenuous—between an experiencing subject and an experienced object. A genuine loving relationship, especially at the height of its sexual expression, approximates this condition of subject-object transcendence. But it only *approximates* it. For this condition of near-genuine love to turn into genuine love, the lovers' images of each other (and of themselves) would have to be sacrificed. In other words, it is only when they come to love the whole person that they love perfectly. And by "whole person" I mean the human being in his or her entirety, comprising both the visible aspects and the invisible dimension; as a manifestation of the Whole (or God) and as that unmanifest Whole itself.

To put it in Hindu terms, perfect love is the love between Shiva and Shakti, between the tranquil, abiding aspect of the Whole (conceived as masculine) and its dynamic counterpart (conceived as feminine). God Shiva and Goddess Shakti—there is much instruction to be found in this kind of mythological imagery—are eternally in blissful embrace or surrender to one another. That is to say, the Absolute or Divine Reality is its own sacrifice: It is both Being *and* Becoming, State *and* Process.

It is in this transcendental condition that we have the key to the surrender which spiritual seekers cultivate. They adopt and follow a path that attempts to "reverse" such normal human values and attitudes as greed, hatred, envy, jealousy, or fearful avoidance. Through this yogic or spiritual "reversal," they create for themselves a life which is analogous to the Divine. Their entire life is modelled on the nonordinary, nonhuman Reality. It becomes an "imitation" (in the best sense of the word) of the milieu of Reality. This is exactly what is implied in Jesus' admonition: "Be perfect, therefore, as your heavenly Father is perfect" (Matthew 5:48). In the same spirit, Saint Paul said: "I have been crucified with Christ, and it is no longer I who live but it is Christ who lives in me" (Galatians 2:20).

The Yoga practitioners, then, surrender their "usualness." The more complete and unquestioning this surrender becomes, the nearer they draw to, or rather the more they participate in, the dimension of absolute Reality. Ultimately, they hope to fully and permanently realize their authentic Being, which is the Self (*atman*).

Next, let me briefly examine the second focus of this essay: faith. The word itself is derived from the Latin term *fides* which means "trust" or "certainty." The first observation to be made is that faith and belief, though frequently thrown into the same pot, denote essentially distinct inner processes. "I believe in God (or the abominable snowman)" means something quite different from "I have faith in God (but not in the Yeti)." Belief is the intellectual judgement that something is such-and-such. It can range from a hypothetical opinion to a deeply held conviction.

Faith is more than that. It is a *radical openness* of oneself to something (or someone) that one considers of superlative personal significance. One of the great theologians of our day, Paul Tillich, described faith as "the state of being grasped by an ultimate concern." In this sense, faith is part of daily life. There is no one who has no faith. True, the object of a person's faith—his or her "ultimate concern"—may be a most unworthy thing, as when a blindly loving wife "worships" a husband who chronically mistreats her.

Faith has to do with the very depths of one's being. It is the mainspring of one's will to live, one's primary inspiration. Therefore when we are in the throes of a "crisis of faith" we experience a profound disorientation and even fear of annihilation. Just like love, as understood above, faith is not simply an emotion. Rather it is a kind of basic orientation within us—a person's "trajectory"—which can become associated with different emotions. Love, again, is a movement of one's whole being toward overcoming the separation between beings. [1]

The spiritual significance of faith and surrender, then, is that both are deeply felt *responses* to something that exceeds our personal life. They well up within us, coming from untold depths, and through them we can consciously reach those very depths.

§

This second section is dedicated to showing how faith and surrender are present in the practice of all the limbs of Yoga.

The foundation of any authentic yogic approach is moral discipline or *yama* (lit., "restraint"). This is meant to regulate the spiritual practitioners' social behavior. Moral integrity is a must for the *yogins* and *yoginis* who do not wish to fall prey to any attitudes and habits that countermand their spiritual aspirations. Through the universal application of the rules of *yama,* they ensure that they will never abuse the power—whether psychic or social—that is acquired in Yoga.

There are five such rules. The root of all of them is said to be "non-harming" (*ahimsa*). This Sanskrit word is also frequently translated as "nonviolence." It consists in one's unconditional non-maliciousness toward all beings at all times and in all situations. *Ahimsa* has to be practiced not only in deed, but also in word and in thought. Thus it includes refraining from gossip and even thinking ill of a person, a whole group of people (e.g., xenophobia, racism, etc.), or even animate beings in general (i.e., speciesism). This presupposes a considerable degree of detachment or "dispassion" (*vairagya*), which, as readers of the *Yoga-Sutra* will know, is one of the two poles of Yoga practice—the other being constant application (*abhyasa*) to the practical disciplines.

How can *ahimsa* be said to be an expression of surrender and faith? The faith component in it is found in the recognition that our authentic Being, the Self, is beyond hurt (*a-himsa*), beyond ill (*an-amaya*), beyond sorrow (*a-duhkha*), beyond pain (*a-klesha*). This being our true nature, we may surrender to it by acknowledging the Self in all other beings and by treating them not as potential or actual enemies but as that universal benign Self.

The virtue of "nonharming," then, is grounded in the recognition that there is no cause for fear with regard to anybody or anything, since all is that same Reality, that same singular Self. Once we have overcome this fundamental fear, which is conjured up by the ego experiencing itself as an island apart from others, we also will be able to practice "nonharming" with consummate skill.

The second constituent of the category of *yama* is "truthfulness" (*satya*). Here the traditional scriptures again demand of us that we cultivate this virtue in action, speech, and thought. The *yogins* or *yoginis* who practice "truthfulness" in this way cannot possibly be prone to lying, hypocrisy, or self-deception. It is easy to see how this virtue is rooted in the moral principle of "nonharming."

Our faith in truthfulness is our faith in Truth, also called *satya*. And Truth is another name for the Self. The Self is that in which there is not a single trace of falsehood; it is the Real, or *tattva*, which literally means "that-ness." Another term for it is *tathata* or "thus-ness," which underscores its *true* nature.

In surrendering to this Truth, we are capable of casting off all the needless ballast of little or big deceptions that people tend to carry around with them all their lives. Again, there is an element of fear-lessness involved in this commitment to Truth (and truths). Even when one has just started to cultivate this virtue, one quickly realizes to what extent our whole civilization is operating on the reverse principle of untruth: from advertising and political campaigning (both of which are almost wholly institutionalized forms of lying), to the manipulation of the law and of "facts" by lawyers, as well as all the myriads of techniques employed by people in order to pre-serve "face" or to remain "one up."

The third component of *yama* is "nonstealing" (*asteya*). Once again, this is to be understood in a very comprehensive sense. As a form of "dispassion" it is the abstention—in deed, word, and thought—from "grasping" after another's property. Even merely coveting our neighbor's strawberries, let alone his wife or her hus-band (who is of course not property), constitutes an infringement of this moral commandment.

This ideal is connected on the one hand with "nongrasping" (*aparigraha*) and on the other hand with "contentment" (*samtosha*), which will be discussed below. Where does faith come into play in this case? The Yoga practitioners' faith is placed in the Self as the inexhaustible Fullness (*purnatva*) that, once it has been realized, leaves nothing to be desired.

Our external grasping after, or seizing of, things (and also relationships) is an expression of the ego's strategy to overcome its basic fearfulness created by its self-isolation (or isolation from the Self). But in this endeavor to extend its radius the ego necessarily encroaches on the life-space of others, and this violates the first law of "nonharming." Through surrender to the Self as the absolutely self-sufficient Reality, the ego's harmful activity is gradually neutralized. The *yogins* or *yoginis* who live this ideal are no longer at war with the world—or themselves.

The next element of *yama* is "chastity" (*brahmacarya*). The literal meaning of this old Sanskrit word is "brahmic conduct," that is, the "behavior of a brahmin" or the "mode of the Absolute." Here the principle of reversal, spoken of above as the very essence of the yogic process, is most clearly expressed. To behave like the Absolute means to model one's life on the ideal condition of the genderless Absolute. This is the underlying idea of "chastity." Our ordinary world-experience is always framed in terms of male and female (and occasionally neuter). "Chastity" is, first of all, the attempt to break away from this binary compartmentalization of life. True continence begins in the mind.

The spiritual practitioners who have mastered this virtue regard all people as "the same" (*sama*)—irrespective of their sex. On the physical level, "chastity" involves the abstinence from sexual activity. Some schools make this an unqualified condition, whereas others hold a more lenient view. The latter apply the principle of moderation to this aspect of one's personal life, but also have rather definite notions about what is to be considered as legitimate sex. Sexual exploitation between men and women, which is often what today's "sexual revolution" is about, is in yogic terms not only a waste of precious life energy (*ojas*), but also a kind of violence, theft, and deception.

Through their faith that the eternal Self not only transcends all bodily distinctions but that it is also inherently blissful (*ananda*), the

Yoga practitioners surrender their desire for the transient pleasure afforded through sexual activity. [2]

The fifth and last member of *yama* is "nongrasping" or "greedlessness" (*aparigraha*). In a way, this is the perfect form of "nonstealing." When everything has been recognized as being alien to one's true Being, then all self-assertion, however subtle, becomes theft. People fall, roughly speaking, into two psychological types. There are those who have what is called "belonging identity" and those who have "awareness identity." [3] To the former, the Yoga practitioner's total disinterest in worldly things (including titles, positions, etc.) will seem either perfectly insane or very frightening. However, to the latter the yogic way of life will make sense more readily. The practitioners of Yoga themselves belong to this second category.

The travelers on the yogic path place their faith in the Self, the ultimate unit of Awareness, which is without properties or qualifications and which is yet the foundation of all things. If they can surrender to it, all avarice will automatically fall away from them.

We now come to the second "limb," the fivefold category of "self-restraint" (*niyama*). Whereas the rules of *yama* are designed primarily to harmonize the Yoga practitioners' social relationships, the disciplines of *niyama* serve to deepen their orientation toward the ultimate Reality.

The first component of *niyama* is "purity" (*shauca*). Often interpreted as mere bodily cleanliness, this practice actually entails much more. From one point of view, the whole yogic path represents itself as an extensive process of purification or catharsis. To paraphrase one of Patanjali's aphorisms (*viz.*, III.55): When the deepest level of one's personality (the *sattva*) is as translucent as the Self, this is equivalent to the condition of liberation.

According to Yoga philosophy the ordinary person lives in a state of corruption or impurity caused by the delusion that he or she is other than the Self, that he or she is a particular body-mind dissociated from the universal Ground of all things, which is simple and devoid of defects. *Shauca* is the gradual retrieval of that essential purity at the innermost core of our being and of the world at large.

Shauca comprises physical cleansing techniques, which came to be especially developed in *hatha-yoga*, but also internal practices intended to remove the cobwebs of the mind. Through *shauca*, so Patanjali tells us (*viz.*, II.40), we acquire a sense of distance from the body. This is the attitude of "dispassion" applied to our most immediate "environment," the body-mind. The Yoga students' faith is in the Self as the eternally pure principle beyond all defects and blemishes. On surrendering to That, they find the inner strength to cease "polluting" their environment, their microcosm, with spiritually marred and hence "impure" actions, words, and thoughts.

The next constituent of *niyama* is "contentment" (*samtosha*). Vyasa, in his commentary on the *Yoga-Sutra* (II.32), explains that this is the "nonhankering after more than is at hand through one's spiritual practice." The attitude behind this is identical with the message contained in the saying attributed to Jesus: "Behold the birds of the air; they neither sow nor reap nor gather into barns, and yet your heavenly Father feeds them" (Matthew 6:26). In other words, the Yoga practitioners "seek first the Kingdom of Heaven" and put their trust in the plenitude of the omnipresent Reality. They surrender their fear that, unless they seize and hoard things, they will not survive. Some of the greatest masters have demonstrated the viability of this principle of contentment by living the simplest life imaginable, while happily passing on to others the wealth and property gifted to them by their disciples.

"Austerity" (*tapas*), the next member of *niyama*, consists in special practices that are meant to test and strengthen our will. Typical exercises are fasting, prolonged sitting, and observing silence. The word *tapas* means literally "heat" or "glow." All *tapas* is a symbolic re-enactment of the *tapas* involved in the creation of the universe. For, according to Hindu mythology (and many other mythologies), the Creator heated himself and sweated out the world.

The yogic *tapas*, however, is practiced for the opposite purpose, namely to resolve the personal universe, our microcosm, back into the single Reality. *Tapas* is thus the surrender or sacrifice of our continual out-flowing tendency, and is founded in our faith in the Absolute as the supreme Power, the ultimate Light.

The fourth element of *niyama* is "self-study" (*svadhyaya*), both in the sense of "study of oneself" and in the sense of "studying by oneself." Vyasa defined it in this way: "*Svadhyaya* is the study of the sciences of liberation and it is [also] the recitation of the *pranava* [i.e., the sacred syllable *om*]." From this explanation it is clear that study does not stand for just any kind of learning. It refers specifically to the Yoga practitioner's consideration of the spiritual heritage of his or her tradition. Perhaps a more liberal view would be to include *all* traditions and, indeed, all forms of knowledge, on the basis that the truly committed Yoga practitioner will be able to extract important lessons from any kind of knowledge, secular and sacred.

The meditative recitation of *om,* or other similar words of power (*mantra*), also leads to spiritually important experiences and insights about the structure of the body-mind. Any form of meditation is, in the last analysis, a means of such self-study.

Where do we find a place for faith and surrender in this practice? Here the spiritual practitioners sacrifice their mind's natural penchant for spiritually insignificant thoughts and subjects, all the futile learning for the mere sake of it. They discipline themselves by resorting to a careful diet of wholesome intellectual "food." Their trust is in the Self as the all-knowing Reality, which is the foundation of all information and which yet transcends all information.

The last component of *niyama* to be explained is "devotion to the Lord" (*ishvara-pranidhana*). While the previous practice addressed our mental capacity, "devotion to the Lord" is a matter of the heart, or feeling. There is no need to interpret this requirement in a narrowly theistic sense. In Classical Yoga the concept of the "Lord" (*ishvara*) is anyway somewhat peculiar and problematic. Perhaps the least complicated way of understanding the present practice is by regarding it as a radical opening up of oneself toward that which is sensed to be greater than oneself.

It is not necessary to think of this Something in terms of a Creator-God. So, even self-styled atheists, provided they appreciate the fact of their own relative insignificance and dependence in the cosmos, can fruitfully embark on this opening-up. Ultimately, this is what has to happen anyway, if the personality is to be transmuted and the ego transcended. The surrender and faith aspects in this practice or attitude are self-evident.

We have now reached the third "limb," the one with which Western students are most familiar, namely "posture" (*asana*). The surrender element in this practice is apparent from Patanjali's instruction (*viz.*, II.47) that "posture," in addition to being firm and comfortable, should be accompanied by the "relaxation of tension" (*prayatna-shaithilya*) as well as "(mental) coinciding with the infinite" (*ananta-sampatti*). "Posture" is thus a letting-go, a loosening-up of the naturally contracted condition of the body-mind. When performed properly, any *asana* turns into a bodily and mental act of expansion.

In performing an *asana*, practitioners surrender their egoic image and experience of the body as something solid with definite boundaries. Thereby they overcome their mistaken notion that the body-mind (in its contracted state) is their authentic nature. The faith expressed in this technique is their trust in the incorporeal (*asharira*) Self that is nonetheless omnipresent.

By means of *pranayama*, the fourth limb, students of Yoga further experience the body as a non-solid, as an energy field. *Prana* is the life energy whose physical manifestation is the breath. *Ayama* means literally "extension," so that *pranayama* signifies the "extension of the life force" by way of controlling and regulating its flow in the body. Patanjali states (*viz.*, II.52) that through this exercise, the "coverings" that conceal the Light within are removed. In this practice the Yoga practitioners place their trust in the universal principle of life, the Self. What they surrender is the ego-bound, disharmonious "energy field," which is their contracted body.

The fifth limb of the eightfold path is "sense-withdrawal" (*pratyahara*). This is the abstraction of the senses from the external world. It is the first proper phase in the cultivation of inwardness leading to concentration and meditation proper. In this exercise the habitual "centrifugal" tendency of consciousness is checked. The attractions of sights and sounds are neutralized so that inner seeing and hearing can develop. The classical texts employ the simile of a tortoise that draws its limbs back into the shell.

Pratyahara is on the sensory level what "nontaking" is on the ethical level. In *pratyahara*, the spiritual practitioners sacrifice their craving for multiplicity so that they may come to realize the One that underlies everything. Their faith is directed to the inner Self, or *pratyag-atman,* which is the Self of all beings and which, in the words of the *Shvetashvatara-Upanishad* (III.19), "sees without eyes, hears without ears."

With "concentration" (*dharana*), the practitioners move out of the sphere of the so-called outer limbs (*bahir-anga*) into the sphere of the "inner limbs" (*antar-anga*) of the eightfold path. Concentration is *asana* applied to the mind. It is a firm, steady focusing of one's consciousness upon a particular internal object or locus within the body. It is the flip side of "sense-withdrawal." Another name for it is "one-pointedness" (*ekagrata*).

In this practice, the spiritual practitioners endeavor to be as single-minded as the One (*eka*) beyond all duality. They surrender their usual identification with the mind's hectic activity. This is expressive of their faith in the Self as that which is beyond the pale of thought and which is yet the basis of all thinking.

The seventh limb of the classical yogic path is "meditation" (*dhyana*). This is a deepened state of concentration in which the same object is held unwaveringly for a long period. It is a more complete form of the practitioner's surrender of his or her mind. It is no longer a mental effort, but a state of reposing in a noncontracted condition of the body-mind. This condition is beautifully described in a passage in the ancient *Chandogya-Upanishad* (VII.6.1) where we can read: "Meditation certainly is more than thought (*citta*). The Earth meditates as it were; the atmosphere meditates as it were . . ." That is to say, meditation is abiding in one's natural state, without mental complications.

The practitioners of Yoga surrender their mind's tendency to appropriate different objects, whether external or internal. Instead they trust in the Self as the Experiencer of all, the Continuity behind the incessant change of the finite world.

The last limb of the eightfold path is *samadhi,* which is generally rendered as "ecstasy." The world-renowned historian of religion Mircea Eliade has proffered an alternative rendering—"enstasy." This coinage takes into account that *samadhi* is not so much a state of exuberance, as suggested by the word "ecstasy," but a condition of great stillness and focusedness in which we "stand in" (*en stasis*) our true nature.

The previously described techniques of concentration and meditation cause a slowing down of the movement within the mental world. In the state of *samadhi,* our inner architecture can be said to collapse altogether. For, the practitioner surrenders the characteristic feature of human consciousness, which is its bi-polar nature, its tension between subject and object. In *samadhi,* the experiencing subject *becomes* the contemplated object.

At the highest level of this paradoxical condition, the experiencer is *all* objects, the entire universe, because it has become the transcendental Self; or rather, the practitioner awakens to the truth that "he" or "she" was the Self all along. The faith element in this process can be said to be the Yoga practitioner's complete trust in the Absolute as pure Awareness.

It is important to understand that the abolition of the ordinary consciousness does not signal a state of unconsciousness or stupor. On the contrary, the Reality revealed in the highest degree of *samadhi* is pure Awareness or *cit.* Or, as the Vedanta scriptures phrase it, it is Being-Consciousness-Bliss (*sat-cid-ananda*).

The Yoga practitioner's recovery of the ultimate Reality, or Self-realization, is the fulfillment of his or her consistently cultivated disposition of faith and surrender. This Self-remembering is perfect self-forgetfulness, which transcends all categories of the mind, including faith and surrender. Faith and surrender call for an object, but for the person who has awakened as the ultimate Reality there is no "outside," no "other." Hence Janaka, upon having been granted the vision of the Absolute by the grace of the enlightened adept Ashtavakra, exclaimed in ecstasy:

> Oh, even among a multitude of people, I see no duality. [Everything is singular] like a closed forest. Upon what should I fix my desire?
>
> Marvelous! In me, the unbounded ocean, [countless] waves of being (*jiva*) come in conflict, play, and merge according to their nature. [4]

Giving testimony to his own realization, Ashtavakra said:

> I am boundless like space; the created universe is like a jar [filled and surrounded by space]. Hence there is no [need for] relinquishing, accepting, or dissolving this [world]. Such is wisdom (*jnana*).
>
> Where is darkness or light, where cessation? Indeed, where is anything at all for the sage who is ever immutable and untroubled?

There is no heaven and no hell, not even living liberation (*jivan-mukti*). In brief, nothing [that could be grasped by the mind presents itself] to the yogic vision. [5]

That which is left when the mind has been stripped of all erroneous ideas about reality is indescribable. It is not a mere void, and, as Ashtavakra and all the other sages vouchsafe, "it" is incomparably blissful.

NOTES

1. I owe this particular insight to Professor Tillich. See his *The Courage to Be* (New Haven, CT: Yale University Press, 1952).

2. See essay 20 for a discussion of the employment of sexual energies in certain schools of Tantrism.

3. This distinction was made by Adam Curle in his book *Mystics and Militants: A Study of Awareness, Identity, and Social Action* (London: Tavistock Publications, 1972).

4. *Ashtavakra-Samhita* II.21 and 25.

5. *Ibid.,* VI.1; XVIII.78, 80.

11

TALKING WITH YOGA MASTER PATANJALI

The following is an imaginary dialogue with the Yoga adept Patanjali who lived sometime in the second century A.D. His aphorisms on Yoga—the *Yoga-Sutra*—have provided me with some of the finest insights into the human condition. More than that, his Sanskrit work has furnished me with countless hours of scholarly reflection, the fruits of which are embodied in several books. This essay is my way of saying thank you and *namas te* to one of the great Yoga masters of all time.

Master Patanjali, may I begin by saying how grateful I am for being granted this interview. I value the opportunity to put some questions to you that, I am sure, many practitioners of Yoga will appreciate having answered by you.

Om.

For almost two thousand years, yogins have celebrated your work as the vade-mecum *of Yoga philosophy and practice. What prompted you to compose the* Yoga-Sutra?

Before I answer your question, let me say that it is gratifying to see modern people, especially Westerners, taking an interest in the age-old tradition of Yoga. It is good to witness the revival of this ancient discipline in the present era. It is also very important, because times are critical. Humanity has maneuvered itself into a corner. This is the Dark Age, the *kali-yuga*, prophesied in our scriptures. The spiritual spark is barely alive in modern men and women, and it must be rekindled and fanned to burn brightly again if humanity is to survive the obstacles that now lie in its path. Science and technology cannot ensure the survival of the human species. In fact, they are mainly responsible for the present situation of skepticism, cynicism, and materialism. Human beings have to change themselves—their approach to life, their very consciousness. They have to take spiritual life and spiritual realities seriously.

If people had indeed celebrated my work, as you say, it would surely not have come to this crisis at all; because when you celebrate something you respect it, and you allow it to influence and transform you. But this hasn't really happened.

Certainly, the *Yoga-Sutra* has changed the course of the development of Yoga, and that is what it was intended to do. You see, in my days, just over seventeen hundred years ago, there were numerous Yoga schools, but there was not a single authoritative voice for the Yoga tradition as a whole. There were many wise and accomplished spiritual teachers, but their teachings were drowned in the cacophony of philosophical disputations. There were the doctors of logic, the teachers of Vedic ritualism, the numerous proponents of nondualism, the metaphysicians of Samkhya, the materialists, and the skeptics—yes, we had our share of them, too. Then there were the Buddhists and the Jainas and other non-Hindus.

The debate was not always fought fairly or objectively, to say the least. Proponents of one system would defend their point of view by misquoting or misrepresenting the opponent's school of thought, just like today. There was, therefore, a real need for authoritative expositions summarizing the position of each school. These statements had to be succinct enough to be memorized, because, as you know, writing was not yet a primary form of communication.

So, the leading authorities of a particular school or tradition did what before them had been tested and found useful by our grammarians: They composed short aphorisms, or word chains, epitomizing the salient aspects of their tradition. Thus, Jaimini created the *Mimamsa-Sutra*, Badarayana the *Brahma-Sutra*, Kanada the *Vaisheshika-Sutra*, Akshapada the *Nyaya-Sutra*, and Kapila the *Samkhya-Sutra*. I rendered a similar service for the Yoga tradition.

Master Patanjali, you mentioned the Samkhya-Sutra *of Kapila. This scripture is nowadays thought to be of a relatively recent date,*

c. *1500* A.D. *However, we know of references to earlier aphorisms that clearly belong to the Samkhya school of thought. Is your own work the only one of its kind, or were there other* sutra-*compilations for the Yoga tradition?*

There were indeed other *Yoga-Sutras,* but for some reason these were not destined to become as widely known as my own work. In fact, I myself adopted a whole group of aphorisms from an earlier composition—those dealing with the eight "limbs" of Yoga. I notice with some dismay that the current version of my work contains a number of distortions and unacceptable additions that were presumably made by my disciples, copyists, and later commentators.

Master Patanjali, which of the Sanskrit commentaries that have been composed to explain your work would you consider most faithful to your original intention?

In his famous commentary, the *Yoga-Bhashya* (III.6), Vyasa cites an old saying: "By Yoga, Yoga must be known; through Yoga, Yoga advances. He who cares for Yoga, In Yoga rests forever." This is absolutely true. The key to understanding Yoga is actual practice of the disciplines of Yoga—the eight limbs. This truth is recognized by all esoteric traditions. It cannot be otherwise. For the ordinary person does not have the depth and range of experience, or the acuity of discernment, necessary to understand the real significance and the inner workings of Yoga.

And yet, how few of those who have commented on my work have taken this piece of wisdom seriously! Vyasa was most certainly a practitioner. So was Shankara who, in his younger days before becoming a spokesman for Vedanta, composed a fine commentary entitled *Vivarana.* However, it must be stated that neither Vyasa nor Shankara practiced according to the way that I taught Yoga. So, we must expect some discrepancies between their interpretations and my original intentions. On the whole, however, their understanding of the *Yoga-Sutra* is correct and definitely helpful.

The later commentators are perhaps less reliable insofar as they deviate from the explanations of Vyasa and Shankara. I wish my own commentaries had survived! I gave extensive notes on the *Yoga-Sutra* to some of my disciples. Some were written down, most were memorized, but all were seemingly lost. As for modern schol-arship, well . . .

If only scholars would find their way to approach Yoga in the same experimental spirit that they apply to the study of Nature! The trouble is that scholars tend to worship the idol of objectivity. They fear to extend their method to the realm of personal experience because they fail to realize that the mind is just as "objective" or "subjective" as atoms, molecules, and inanimate objects. The mind, or *citta,* is a manifestation of Nature, and its functioning can be in-vestigated with the same acuteness as any other phenomenon. In fact, many aspects of Nature will remain hidden until the mind is better understood. By controlling the mind, *yogins* develop special psychic capacities, which give them more direct knowledge of the subtle dimensions of Nature that are as yet closed to science. In some respects, the "subjective" approach of Yoga is superior to the "objective" orientation of science. I think the glorification of objec-tivity is entirely whimsical.

If scholars and scientists were to practice the higher stages of Yoga, they soon would be convinced of the primacy of Awareness (*cit*). Typically, scientists confine themselves to a narrow range of approaches to reality. Their search for truth can be severely limited by their exclusive faith in the lower mind, or *manas.* They tend to shun the higher intuitions and perceptions of the person who has transformed his or her consciousness through spiritual disciplines. And in doing so, they end up ignoring a vast body of reality. Yoga is a means of understanding and experiencing the psychophysical na-ture of reality, which goes beyond the material cause-and-effect universe. It permits the practitioner to acquire firsthand knowledge of the inconceivable complexity of the universe, which science is finally beginning to admit.

But Yoga is not merely an alternative science or a superscience. It is first and foremost a method of *spiritual transformation* to the point where the world is transcended, where the human being re-covers his or her essential nature as the transcendental Awareness, which I call *purusha.* So, the purpose of Yoga is to guide us beyond all experience, beyond all knowledge, beyond all forms of belief, beyond all questions and answers. [*Patanjali chuckles*]

*Master Patanjali, if you were to write a summary of the Yoga tra-
dition today, would you choose the medium of aphorisms, or* sutras,
again?

Obviously not. People's memories have deteriorated just like
their eyesight. The printed word has been a blessing and a curse,
like so many of modern humanity's inventions. The aphoristic style
was appropriate for the purposes I had in mind, and for that time.
Today a different kind of communication is required. But what I had
to say in my work is still essentially valid.

There *is* a transcendental Reality that is our inmost nature. That
Reality is pure Awareness, or *cit*, without content or form. It is beyond all change and infinite. The body-mind is simply a product of
the transient aspect of Nature, or *prakriti*. The body-mind is not our
true identity. The finite body-mind is something we assume ourselves to be, owing to our spiritual ignorance. It springs from our
spiritual blindness and gives rise to the whole host of complications
that characterize people's unenlightened lives.

Yoga is a practical discipline to end this false identification with
the body-mind and to restore us to our true nature—as the transcendental Self, the *purusha*. The efficacy of Yoga as a technique of
liberation has been demonstrated by many adepts. It is universally
applicable because human nature is essentially the same everywhere. The Yoga tradition has grown in richness since the days
when I composed the *Yoga-Sutra*, but these developments have not
changed the principles that make Yoga the effective tool that it is.

*Master Patanjali, your philosophy has been described as strictly
dualistic, because you oppose the principle of Awareness, or the*
purusha, *to the principle of materiality, or* prakriti. *This sort of duality
is adamantly denied by all the nondualist traditions of India. Who
has the correct interpretation of reality?*

[*Laughs*] All interpretations of reality are equally one-sided. If
you argue that there is only one principle and that everything else
is merely an illusion, then you are obviously achieving this
nonduality by sacrificing the evidence of your senses. On the other
side, if you argue that there are two chief principles—Awareness

and materiality—then you create this duality on the basis of the limited understanding that arises from sensory experience.

The danger of the former interpretation is that it can turn into rampant idealism combined with an emotional alienation from the world. This can be seen in many of the ascetic schools of India. It can also give rise to an attitude of hypocrisy, whereby a mere believer in the truth of nonduality may behave as if he or she had realized that singular Reality, which they call *atman* or *brahman*. It would seem that many contemporary adherents of nondualism have actually fallen prey to this delusion.

I have chosen a dualistic framework precisely because it avoids that particular fallacy. I felt that dualism reflects more adequately the condition of the seeker after truth, and is therefore also more conducive to spiritual practice. In fact, all spiritual discipline is essentially dualistic: On one side, there is the spiritual practitioner, and on the other side, there is the Reality toward which the practitioner aspires. There is the transcendental Awareness, and there is the whole configuration of his or her body-mind that must be purified and transformed.

Unfortunately, my position has not always been fully understood. If you examine my work carefully, you will discover that there is not a single statement that would bear out the kind of strict dualist philosophy that is generally attributed to me. I suggest that modern scholars have been misled by earlier commentators on this point. With all the seers and sages who have glorified my homeland by their wisdom, I affirm that there is only one Truth, one Reality, and that this reality is pure Awareness. I have given that Awareness the name *cit*, *cit-shakti*, or *purusha*.

I am not interested in discussing whether what we perceive as material Nature, or *prakriti*, is illusory or real from the absolute point of view. What matters is that materiality is real for the practitioner who is still on his or her journey of discovery, who has not yet realized the ultimate Being, who is not yet liberated. In this respect I am a thorough pragmatist.

Master Patanjali, what about the moral requirements, the yamas *and* niyamas? *Are they still applicable today? There are those who argue that this kind of ethical code has become obsolete and is no longer useful in the context of our modern civilization.*

Such people couldn't be more mistaken! The rules of *yama* and *niyama* have of course always been unpopular. There never was a right time for them! [*Chuckles*] People have always looked for an excuse not to practice them. Truthfulness (*satya*), for instance, is certainly not useful in a culture where deceit is the rule. Look at your advertising, which is built on deliberate distortions. Look at the mass media, which are communicating such a lopsided view of reality that they can be said to cultivate the untruth. And so on.

What about nonharming (*ahimsa*)? Well, your civilization is undoubtedly the most violent that ever existed. You have to lock your front doors and peep through spy-holes before you allow a visitor into your homes. You cannot even walk safely in your big cities anymore. Husbands batter wives, and parents abuse their children, while youngsters mug the old who are anyway treated like outcastes. You have fought two world wars in this century alone and waged several hundred smaller but nevertheless equally harmful wars.

And you are constantly living on the brink of a third world war, which, as you all sense, would probably obliterate the human population and render this planet inhospitable for a long time to come. Some of your finest apostles of nonviolence—Gandhi and Martin Luther King—were rewarded for their peacemaking efforts by being assassinated. Wouldn't you say that your civilization could do with a dose of nonharming?

You speak of your society as a consumer society. Tens of thousands of factories turn out a never-ending stream of goods designed to lull hundreds of millions of people into a false sense of comfort. But those who can afford these goods and services generally do not give a thought to the fact that there are many more millions who are literally starving. While the wealthy, industrialized nations ransack the earth's resources to increase their citizens' standard of living— but also their ill-health and sense of unfulfillment—one third of humanity lives in abject poverty. This is shortsighted politically as well as deeply unjust—a clear instance of theft. Cluttering up your life with possessions that are not essential to your personal welfare, while some people still go hungry, is literally stealing. As the Yoga masters of old taught and as your modern physicists have rediscovered, Nature is a great ecological system that, sooner or later, redresses any imbalance. Be warned, therefore!

The secret of all the wisdom traditions lies in nongrasping (*aparigraha*), in not expecting Nature to be your salvation or fulfillment. Nothing in Nature can ultimately fulfill you. Nothing in Nature can give you lasting happiness, enduring bliss, or permanent freedom. This holds true today as it did two thousand years ago. Only the transcendental Awareness is sheer, unalloyed bliss.

Your civilization is obsessed with sex, as were many other cultures in the past. Why? Because you seek to capture some of that ultimate, lasting bliss in the midst of a frenetic existence whose basic mood is stress. You are basically unhappy people, seeking relief from chronic tension. For most people, sex affords a semblance of happiness—however momentary. The thrill of orgasm is only a poor substitute for the supreme ecstasy of Self-realization.

Don't you think that the old-fashioned moral virtue of chastity (*brahmacarya*) in thought, word, and deed would be a real advantage to your civilization? One doesn't need to be a puritan to appreciate that chastity is a useful discipline in a cultural environment that degrades men and women by fostering values and attitudes that promote a kind of mechanical sexuality divorced from all emotion.

I would say, unless your civilization succeeds in realizing the virtues embodied in the *yamas* and *niyamas*, its outlook is more than bleak.

Master Patanjali, people nowadays have great difficulty in applying themselves to a spiritual discipline. You indicated in the Yoga-Sutra *that the yogic path is an arduous and a prolonged affair. Most people are obliged to work long hours every day to earn their livelihood, and so they are not able to pursue spiritual practice with the necessary energy and endurance . . .*

[*Interrupts*] Their dilemma is not new! It is the householder's eternal difficulty. Today, circumstances are considerably different from those of yore—at least externally. The real problem, though, hasn't changed one bit. The question is always: What are your priorities? Do you want to invest your energy and attention in making a successful material life for yourself and your family, or do you want to throw yourself with your whole being into the fire of spiritual life? Most people are too lethargic even to pose this fundamental question seriously. Many remain dilettantes, dabblers in spiritual life.

From nine to five they are cool business men and women, five or six days a week. And then, for perhaps an hour in the evening, provided that they don't feel too stressed out or tired, they seek to reduce their discomfort by meditating. Mostly, they don't aspire to more than that. I hope I am not being too harsh. Also, I am not saying that what they are doing is wrong or worthless. Meditation, even at this level, is a useful instrument, and they may well reduce their stress and blood pressure. They may even become better people.

But the principal purpose of spiritual life is not to feel more relaxed or to be merely happier and healthier. Rather, spiritual life is about cultivating the intuition of one's true identity, the Self. It is about not being caught up in the tendency to identify with a particular body-mind, environment, or circumstance. And that is a practice that needs to be fostered throughout the day in all one's activities.

Master Patanjali, in reading the Yoga-Sutra *I have always been struck by the fact that the devotional element, or* bhakti, *is not given much prominence. This has led people to contrast your teaching with the* bhakti-yoga *of the* Bhagavad-Gita *and other similar scriptures. What role does human emotion and especially love-devotion play in your teaching?*

Emotions, like thoughts, are merely agitations of the finite body-mind. They obscure our true nature. The transcendental Awareness is beyond thoughts and emotions and is eternally witnessing all the phenomena arising in the orbit of Nature. Very simply, emotions can be either positive or negative. I have summarized them under the headings of attraction (*raga*) and aversion (*dvesha*). As such they belong to the five causes of suffering, the *kleshas*. The other three *kleshas* are spiritual ignorance, the ego-sense, and the thirst for life.

These form the matrix of human motivation. So long as they are in place, the human being is necessarily oriented toward experiences in the finite realms of Nature. When the *kleshas* are uprooted or burned off, however, there is enlightenment. Liberation. Thus, even seemingly positive emotions like friendship or love are ultimately to be transcended. They pertain to the unenlightened state of the body-mind. Liberated adepts literally transcend good and evil, as I have made clear in my work. They have no *karma*, because they are no longer a particular ego piling up *karma* on themselves through egoic volitions, actions, and emotions.

Master Patanjali, if all emotions belong to the domain of materiality, or Nature, and are foreign to the transcendental Awareness, how is it that some adepts— like Krishna—praise devotion or love (bhakti) *as a superior means of liberation and even as a sign of Self-realization?*

Don't be misled into a futile comparison or search for the only right or true method! Every adept teaches the way that has proven successful in his or her own case. They always impart only what they have tested and fulfilled in their own life. This alone qualifies them to teach and guide others. But there are many ways to Self-realization, just as there are many ways of speaking about the ultimate Reality. Krishna calls it the "Supreme Person" (*purusha-uttama*), the Buddha referred to it as "extinction" (*nirvana*), and I prefer the term "aloneness" (*kaivalya*) for it.

Love or devotion is a powerful force that, if harnessed properly, can indeed carry a practitioner swiftly to liberation. But, like all other methods, it becomes fruitful only when a practitioner has been awakened by an adept who teaches this form of Yoga. You see, initiation in which the adept empowers the practitioner or devotee is essential to all paths. This was clearly understood in ancient times. The *guru* has always been honored as the gateway to liberation.

So, some adepts teach liberation through yoking the body-mind by means of love or devotion. Others guide their devotees to Self-realization by means of renunciation, and yet others by means of the recitation of a *mantra*, or by maintaining a witnessing disposition in active life. These are merely different emphases. My own teaching stresses the control of the mind through meditation and higher contemplation (*samadhi*). But in all approaches, there is an element of yielding or surrendering the false self-sense, the ego, and this could be described as a form of devotional practice.

Master Patanjali, this explanation is very clarifying. If I understand you correctly, what you are implying is that there can be no do-it-yourself Yoga, no home-spun path to Self-realization, but . . .

[*Interrupts*] A torch is lit by another torch. This is what spiritual transmission is all about. There is the realized adept and there is the seeker, the struggling practitioner, who deems himself or herself separate from that which is sought. By virtue of their Self-realization, the adepts initiate in their students a process that will ultimately duplicate their own realization in the aspirant. This is a great Yoga. This is the secret of all the high esoteric traditions. This is what modern seekers must come to understand. The *Shiva-Samhita* (III.1) declares: "Only knowledge that comes from the mouth of a teacher is alive." Although this scripture was composed nearly a millennium and a half after my life on earth, this piece of wisdom is timeless.

Master Patanjali, it appears that your teaching has a strong ascetical orientation, and the spiritual way recommended by you is based on the control of emotions and desires. This contrasts with the path of Tantrism, for instance, where emotions are utilized rather than curbed in the pursuit of spiritual realization. Do you agree with this characterization of your teaching?

Not entirely. It is true that Tantric Yoga represents a different approach to my own. There have always been two main currents in the esoteric traditions of India—one having a more ascetical orientation suitable for renunciates, the other being more accessible to householders. But the ascetical schools were for the most part predominant—and for very good reasons, as I will explain shortly.

At any rate, to contrast these two currents by saying that the ascetical approach is based on the control of emotions whereas the nonascetical approach is not is rather misleading. *All* spiritual paths are founded on the principle of transmuting the ordinary being, and this necessarily entails the transformation of our emotional life.

Tantrism has attracted much bad press, as you would say, in the past and in the present. Why? Because this matter of the deployment of emotions in the ritual Yoga of the Tantras has tended to be grossly misunderstood. Tantrism is *not* hedonism. It is not a materialist philosophy masquerading as a doctrine of salvation. It is not a path of self-fulfillment, but a great way of self-undoing, of self-transcendence, of liberation from the ego-personality. When Tantric practitioners say that liberation (*mukti*) is identical with enjoyment (*bhukti*), then they certainly do not equate the unsurpassable bliss of Self-realization with mere sensory pleasure.

There are those who delude themselves, thinking that because they combine the sexual act with certain Yoga techniques they spiritualize their lust. Yet, whichever way you look at it, orgasm isn't ecstasy. It is a temporary excitation of the nervous system, a rather ephemeral bodily thrill. Still, for the ordinary person, orgasm is the most intense bodily pleasure of which he or she is capable. Other sensory or intellectual stimulations fall far short of the delight of orgasm. But orgasm is not the ultimate delight, or bliss, that is the very essence of Self-realization.

So, obviously, Tantric practitioners must mean something else by the maxim that liberation and enjoyment are not essentially different. In fact, their statement is an *esoteric* utterance. It belongs to the twilight language of Tantrism. As such it is similar to the secret doctrine of *nirvana* being equal to *samsara,* that is to say, the ultimate Reality being equal to the conditional reality; or the Upanishadic teaching that the essence of individuality, the *atman,* is identical with the essence of objective existence, or *brahman.* These are esoteric formulas spoken from the enlightened point of view. They are the ecstatic confessions or testimonies of realized adepts.

So long as you have not actually realized the ultimate Reality, which I choose to call *purusha,* you are still trapped in the limitations of unenlightened existence. Therefore, *samsara* is still *samsara* for you, and enjoyment is not the perfect bliss of Reality but simply enjoyment without any liberating power or grace. What is more, if you were to apply the adept's transcendental wisdom prematurely to your own condition, you would merely court disaster. By confusing your ordinary enjoyments with the extraordinary bliss of Self-realization, you would merely reinforce your enslavement to the sensory realm and thus delay your spiritual liberation.

Lesser practitioners of Tantrism have again and again fallen prey to this lack of discrimination and behaved as if they were enlightened. In effect, they merely indulged themselves and brought

Tantrism into disrepute. Far from bridling their appetites, they let their passions and emotions get the better of them. They allowed themselves to be duped by ignorance rather than guided by *buddhi*, or inspired understanding. They were simply hedonists, not realizers, and their fate necessarily followed the inexorable law of *karma*.

As is made clear in the Tantric scriptures, this particular form of Yoga is not for those who are still ruled by their earthly desires but only for those who are "heroic." In the last chapter of the *Kula-Arnava-Tantra* (XII), the Tantric "hero" (*vira*) is said to be so named because he is free from attachment, intoxication, affliction, anger, jealousy, and delusion. Few practitioners have these virtues to begin with. Therefore, I feel, most are best advised not to experiment with Tantric Yoga. Instead, they should adopt a more ascetical lifestyle. This is, in fact, what the majority of spiritual aspirants throughout the world have done in the past.

And this approach is just as valid today. Human nature hasn't really changed over the past three thousand years, since the time when the foremost of our sages began to espouse asceticism and started to develop methods and techniques that would assist practitioners in their spiritual struggle. It seems to me that the only way in which a person could pursue a nonascetical path with any hope of success is through the graceful agency of a Self-realized adept—and such adepts are exceedingly rare. In other approaches, one's teacher need not necessarily be a fully realized being, though ideally he or she should be. With few exceptions, teachers can take a disciple only as far as they themselves have traveled on the path.

Master Patanjali, in one of your aphorisms (II.38), you state: "When grounded in chastity, vitality is acquired." Is it not also the purpose of ritual intercourse in Tantrism to enhance one's vitality?

That is so. But again, the Tantric ritual of *maithuna* is conducted as a form of spiritual practice that presupposes a chaste mind. It would offer no consolation to a worldly-minded person. Such people always assume that chastity and asceticism turn the *yogin* into an impotent weakling. They fail to notice the shining face of the true ascetic who is continuously transmuting his sexual drive into spiritual energy. Such ascetics are masters of the art of *urdhva-retas*, the upward flow of semen. In this secret practice, the semen is transmuted into subtle energy, called *ojas*, which streams upward into the brain rather than down and out through the genitals.

Genuine sexual sublimation is a psychophysiological process that changes one's body chemistry. It has nothing to do with repression, which only leads to sexual aberration or what you call neurosis. *Urdhva-retas* is essential to the *yogin* who is intent on entering the higher stages of meditative practice. For, the vital energy retained in the nervous system from sexual abstinence—in thought and deed— is a reservoir from which he can draw in order to catapult himself into the condition of ecstasy (*samadhi*). Of course, this holds true of female practitioners as well.

Master Patanjali, you spoke of the bliss of the Self. It always struck me that there is no mention of this aspect of Reality in the Yoga-Sutra.

Reality is without features, without qualities. When the sages of the *Upanishads* praised the bliss (*ananda*) of the Self, they did not mean to ascribe to it any specific quality. That bliss is not a mortal emotion or sensation. It *is* Reality. It *is* the Self. When composing my *Sutra* I chose to de-emphasize this particular teaching, because it can so easily be misunderstood. Instead, I spoke of the Self as pure Awareness (*cit*).

Of course, the ideal way of expressing the transcendental Reality is to remain silent. The Buddha applied himself to this option with consummate skill. But even he was occasionally moved to make concessions to the unillumined mind. The great Buddhist teachers of India, who were my contemporaries, did not in the least shy away from equating Reality with pure Awareness. Neither did I. Indeed, I have been inspired by their teachings. I have even availed myself of some of their concepts and terms to express my own thoughts. Having said this, I hasten to add that I am most certainly not a Buddhist. This will be clear from even a cursory study of my *Sutra*, which should be read with the aid of the old commentaries, especially Vyasa's *Bhashya*.

Master Patanjali, in your Yoga-Sutra *(II.32) you list study* (svadhyaya) *as one of the practices of* niyama. *How important is*

*study? It seems to me that in order to understand your work, mod-
ern practitioners need to have a certain scholastic aptitude.*

That's true enough, but you don't have to be a scholar to comprehend my teaching! To a certain extent, serious practitioners can
rely on the findings of modern scholarship. They don't have to learn
Sanskrit or study for a Ph.D. in Hindu philosophy to understand me,
though it might be a good discipline for some. However, my *Sutra*
was never intended to serve as a do-it-yourself manual for novices,
and it presupposes intimacy with the spiritual culture of my homeland.

Above all, my work can't replace the living wisdom of a teacher.
You cannot go out into the wilderness and hope to practice Yoga
successfully—equipped with only a loincloth and my aphorisms. It
could take you years to discover, for instance, what I meant when I
explained that posture (*asana*) is accompanied by "the relaxation of
tension and coinciding with the infinite" (II.47). An experienced
teacher, however, could show you in seconds what it means to
coincide with the infinite.

Posture would happen spontaneously in such an adept's company, providing he or she has mastered at least this level. When the
practice of posture is accomplished, the body opens up. It begins to
radiate. That radiation is not just a subjective experience. It is a force
that can be felt by others as well. It is as infectious as yawning. But
perhaps that's not a fitting analogy! Posture is a dynamic state, even
though to the outsider you appear to be as immobile as a tree trunk.

Study is essential but actual practice of the moral precepts, posture, breath control, and meditation is equally as important. As the
Vishnu-Purana (VI.6.2–3) declares:

> From study one should proceed to Yoga, and from Yoga to study. By
> perfection in study and Yoga the supreme Self becomes evident.
> Study is one eye to behold That, and Yoga is the other.

*Master Patanjali, are you saying then that intellectual activity is
not a hindrance to Self-realization?*

[*Laughs*] Is this a scholar's bid for the mind? You have studied my
work, so you know that conceptualization (*vikalpa*) is among the

five mental fluctuations to be curbed. I made it clear that this activity of the mind is to be checked even when it appears in the ecstatic state. So, how can it not be a hindrance?

Still, thinking has its place in ordinary functional life. It is even useful in spiritual practice. Thus, this conversation could not occur without *vikalpa*. In the case of an enlightened being, thinking forms itself of its own accord without the intervention of the ego. Therefore it is not a fluctuation in the sense spoken of in my *Sutra*. The awareness of an enlightened being is continuous. It is not interrupted by any mental activity, not even sleep.

In the enlightened condition, all the phenomena of the ordinary consciousness may freely arise, but there is no one to identify with them. Patanjali is not the Patanjali before you. Patanjali is the *purusha*, pure Awareness. It is your mind alone that constructs the sense of egoic individuality both in relation to yourself and to me.

Master Patanjali, with due respect, this sounds like Mahayana Buddhism or Advaita Vedanta. I always assumed that in your teaching, liberation coincides with the dropping of the physical body and that you do not espouse the ideal of liberation while yet alive.

[*Laughs*] That is indeed your assumption, your *vikalpa*.

Well, Master Patanjali, in your work you seem to make a sharp distinction between the principle of Awareness (purusha) *and the principle of materiality* (prakriti). *Your philosophy has for this reason been described as a strict dualism. Now, liberation holds true when there is no longer any identification with the aspects of the material principle. Thus, in the very last aphorism (IV.34), you speak of the "involution"* (pratiprasava) *of the constituents, the gunas, of the universe. That is to say, upon liberation these gunas resolve back into the unmanifest soup of the universe—and this is equivalent to the death of the individual who has become liberated.*

[*Smiles*] So, you made a conjecture! It turns out to be wrong. There is really nothing in my work to justify reading my philosophy as either dualism or monism. I carefully confined myself to speaking about the processes leading up to Self-realization. It is true that I preferred—and still prefer—a framework that brings out the contrast between transcendental Awareness and materiality. But this duality is a relative one, which is simply intended to serve the practical purpose of allowing the practitioner to distinguish, in his or her intuition, between the Real and the unreal. Why assume that liberation coincides with physical death? What *is* involved is the death of the ego, the curious notion of being a subject trapped in a particular body-mind.

Master Patanjali, this sounds strikingly similar to the nondualist philosophy of Vedanta.

Only historians and philosophers are disturbed by similarities. They prefer contrast because contrast can be categorized and labeled. But the spiritual practitioner is not to be troubled by any of this. He or she is to care less for conceptual similarities and dissimilarities than for the underlying experiences and realities. Dualism and nondualism are labels, which may or may not be appropriate and convenient. [*Laughs*] When you are enlightened, everything will be obvious. It's certainly much, much simpler than the mind would have it!

I appreciate what you are saying, Master Patanjali. But may I ask you another question along these lines?

Yes.

In the nondualist tradition of Advaita Vedanta, the transcendental Self, the atman, *is said to be one only. But some authorities maintain that you taught, like the Samkhya school, that there is a transcendental Self, or* purusha, *for each individual . . .*

There are as many opinions as there are individuals. It is all *vikalpa,* a product of the conceptual mind. Nowhere in my work do I speak of multiple Selves. That sounds like schizophrenia. What could multiple Selves possibly be like? There is either infinity and transcendence or there is not. In one of my aphorisms (II. 54), I state that the ultimate realization is "omni-objective," "omni-temporal," and "nonsequential." Now, if that is so—if the crowning realization covers indeed all space and time and is simultaneous—then, how could there be several or many of its kind? Liberation is not an experience. It does not occur to, or within, the mind. It is transcendental. As such, it does not fit any of your categories, and such descriptive labels as singularity and plurality do not apply. So long as such labels can be meaningfully attached to a given condition, that condition necessarily falls short of liberation.

I am not a follower of the Samkhya school of thought. Nor am I a Vedanta philosopher. I am not even a representative of Classical Yoga. I am that Reality upon which all these conceptual categories are projected and in which all these differences seemingly arise.

Master Patanjali, I must confess that this is all a little confusing to me. Do you believe that this differentiated world is an illusion?

Your confusion is due to your philosophical and other presuppositions. As for the illusory nature of the universe, that is the position of Shankara Acarya and his followers. There is a traditional story about Shankara that is pertinent to our consideration. One day, that great teacher was walking down a road when suddenly a mad elephant was stomping toward him at full speed. Shankara wasted no time but ran as fast as his legs would bear him, seeking shelter. Later someone challenged him: "You believe that this world is illusory. Why then did you flee from that elephant?" Shankara promptly replied: "The incident that you witnessed, with the person named Shankara running away from a mad elephant, only occurred in your mind. It was altogether an illusion!"

Now, in all fairness to Shankara, who was a philosophical genius, the story is no more than popular fiction. But it hints at the fact that what from a more subtle, metaphysical point of view may be considered an illusion, can still be experienced as very real. If the event in that anecdote had really happened and if Shankara would have ignored the elephant, he would certainly have been trampled to death.

Thus, there can be no doubt that life and the whole struggle for survival, as experienced by billions of beings, is real as an experience. It would be absurd to deny the reality of, say, your and my body-mind, the blue sky, or the grass on which we sit. That is why I specifically included in my *Sutra* (IV.16) an aphorism that refutes all idealist interpretations.

Yet, what we experience is not the whole truth, is not Reality as it is in itself. Our attention is selective. In fact, it is only when the game of attention is altogether transcended that enlightenment occurs. And then the transcendental Awareness shows itself to be one's true identity. However, the world as experienced by the unillumined mind does not cease to exist upon enlightenment. It continues to bewilder everyone else. Otherwise it would have vanished into thin air with the enlightenment, or liberation, of the very first awakened adept.

What is it then that changes upon liberation, Master Patanjali?

Nothing from the enlightened viewpoint. Everything from the viewpoint of the ego-personality. Look upon life as a dream and upon all so-called sentient beings as actors in that dream. When the great event of liberation occurs there is simply this awakening within the dream. Somehow the dream continues, but the one who is now wide awake witnesses the whole drama without being implicated in it. You will have to awaken yourself to appreciate this truth.

Thank you, Master Patanjali, for your patient instruction.

Om. Peace.

12

THE HISTORY OF HATHA-YOGA

Many Western students of Yoga think that Yoga began in the second century A.D. with Patanjali, author of the *Yoga-Sutra*. But the Yoga tradition is at least seven centuries older than that. In fact, some scholars even discern traces of an archaic Yoga in the ancient Indus civilization, which came to a mysterious and sudden end some four thousand years ago. For their main evidence they point to a terra-cotta seal showing a *yogin*-like figure, which in all likelihood represents a horned deity.

This figure is often identified as a prototype of the later god Shiva Pashupati, the "patron saint" of *hatha-yoga,* whose name means "lord of beasts," lord of all unenlightened beings, fettered by their karmas (or tendencies) to the world of experience like beasts tethered to a tree. This deity is depicted as seated in what could be a yogic posture (*asana*). Such poses, however, are common in representations from antiquity, since chairs (together with hunched shoulders) had not yet been invented. Therefore, the sitting pose of the figure on the seal need not necessarily have any hidden purpose. But one is free to exercise one's historical imagination.

Certainly, given their emphasis on spiritual matters, the Indus people may well have recognized the connection between bodily posture, breath, and mental tranquillity. Yet the complex poses that have become the trademark of *hatha-yoga* are inventions of a much later period, as is the idea of employing them for therapeutic ends.

Originally the term *asana* simply referred to the seat on which the *yogin* would comfortably sink into deep meditation or even swoon in ecstasy. The seat was made of grass, cloth, or the hide of a deer, tiger, or other animal. Later the term came to be applied mainly to the different postures that *yogins* would assume during meditation. This is how it was understood by Patanjali, and also by Vyasa, who wrote the oldest known commentary on the *Yoga-Sutra* in the fifth century.

By the turn of the first millennium A.D., *hatha-yoga* as we know it had already come into its own. Manuals were being compiled that gave a proliferation of postures meant to heal, strengthen, and rejuvenate the body and to prepare it for the challenges of intense and prolonged meditation. With the appearance of *hatha-yoga,* the tradition of Yoga took a new turn.

What had occurred? Nobody knows for sure. The historical evolution of Yoga is exceedingly complex and scantily researched. Moreover, because Yoga is an esoteric tradition that for countless generations was kept alive by word of mouth, the material evidence is relatively scarce. Teachers would pass on their understanding to their disciples, and then, when the disciples had become teachers in their own right, they would do the same with their pupils.

When writing became popular, only the more scholarly minded practitioners of Yoga would write anything down. And even then the real secrets of a particular school continued to be divulged only verbally to initiates. So the scriptures that today form the basis of our understanding of Yoga are more like skeletal treatments than full-bodied sourcebooks.

In the tradition of *hatha-yoga,* the hundred or so manuscripts that survive from different eras give us mostly dry descriptions of practices with sketchy instructions, plus a plenitude of esoteric imagery. Luckily, authentic *hatha-yoga* teachers belonging to one or another established line of adepts do still exist. Thus, what is kept out of books can be learned directly from a living master.

However, most of the history of *hatha-yoga* is lost forever in the timeless mists of ancient India. All we have are a relatively few texts, lists of names of adepts, and very few definite dates. But we do have a multitude of legends about some of the great Yoga masters of antiquity, and some of these stories are popular in India even today.

Many of these tales concern incidents in the lives of two great masters, Goraksha and Matsyendra. Goraksha is celebrated throughout India as the founding father of *hatha-yoga,* and Matsyendra was his teacher and a foremost adept of the Natha tradition.

According to one legend, a woman once implored Shiva, the supreme deity, to grant her a child. Touched by her fervent prayers, Shiva gave her a magical substance to eat. In her ignorance, the woman failed to eat it and instead threw it on a dung heap.

Twelve years later Matsyendra, in the shape of a fish, overheard a secret conversation between Shiva and his divine spouse, Parvati, about the woman's request. Wishing to see the child granted to her by Shiva, Matsyendra went to visit the woman, who confessed to him what had happened. Unperturbed, he asked her to search the dung heap, and—lo and behold!—she found a twelve-year-old boy, whom she named Goraksha.

Matsyendra adopted Goraksha as his disciple, and soon the student's popularity exceeded that of his teacher. In some stories Goraksha is depicted as using his magical powers for the benefit of his teacher.

According to one legend, Matsyendra went to visit Ceylon, where he fell in love with the queen. She invited him to stay with her in the palace, and before long Matsyendra was completely ensnared in worldly life. When Goraksha heard about his teacher's fall, he at once went in search of him and confronted him in the halls of the court. When Matsyendra came to his senses, remembering his former self, he returned to India.

Matsyendra was accompanied by his two sons, Parasnath and Nimnath, adepts in their own right. Later, insists another story, Goraksha killed Matsyendra's sons, only to restore them to life. All these legends, of course, have deep symbolic significance.

Exact dates for Matsyendra and Goraksha are disappointingly (if typically) unknown. According to scholarly consensus, Goraksha lived in the eleventh century and Matsyendra somewhat earlier, though some authorities propose that he was not a historical personage at all. Whatever we know of either of them derives exclusively from folk tradition. "Goraksha" and "Matsyendra" may well have been spiritual appellations bestowed on *yogins* of a particular level of attainment.

The Sanskrit word *goraksha* literally means "protector of cows." *Go* is also one of the secret designations for "passion," and thus *goraksha* suggests someone who has controlled his sexual appetite. Indeed, Goraksha, the adept, is widely remembered as a great ascetic. According to one legend, he turned himself into an innocent babe when a Goddess asked him to marry her, lying in her arms waiting to be suckled.

The name *matsyendra* means "lord of fish." According to esoteric explanations, anyone who carries the title *matsyendra* has mastered the practice of suspending breath and mind through the *khecari mudra*.

This key technique of classical *hatha-yoga* is performed by rolling the tongue back and blocking the air passages of the throat. In most people the tongue does not reach anywhere near the back of the throat, and so *hatha-yoga* recommends a long preparatory practice of "milking" the tongue in order to lengthen it. Those who are skilled in this particular practice can touch at least the tip of the nose with their tongue. In some cases the tongue has been lengthened to reach the place of the "third eye" between the eyebrows.

All kinds of measurable physiological changes occur in the body through regular practice of *khecari-mudra*, the "gesture of moving in space." Here "space" denotes both the cavity at the back of the palate and the infinite ether of transcendental consciousness. The scriptures of *hatha-yoga* abound in such double meanings. Also, this curious practice is said to lead to all kinds of paranormal abilities, including the ability to transfer one's consciousness out of the physical body.

Matsyendra and Goraksha are remembered as supreme masters of this technique. In fact, another meaning of the name *goraksha* is "protector of the tongue." Yet, the principal purpose of such practices was not the attainment of magical powers. Rather, the teachings of both masters were concerned with cultivating the even flow of the life-force (*prana*) circulating in the body so that one might realize the great joy that surpasses the mechanics of mind and nervous system.

The esoteric significance given to the word *hatha* hints at the strictly spiritual orientation of these teachings. The dictionary meaning of *hatha* is "force"; thus *hatha-yoga* is the forceful Yoga, the Yoga that calls for great strength of character and physical stamina. The deeper meaning, however, is that it is the "union" (*yoga*) of *prana* and *apana*, the two main currents of the body's life-force.

The syllable *ha* in *hatha* denotes the solar (right) current, and the syllable *tha* denotes the lunar (left) current. For true well-being, which includes enlightenment, both currents must flow evenly along the central axis of the body.

Matsyendra, Goraksha, and other masters of the Natha tradition contributed to India's spiritual heritage a novel insight into the physiological basis of spiritual practice. As a result, they succeeded in devising techniques that allow the *yogin* to manipulate his energy patterns. Recently the yogic discovery of the body's bipolar energy current has been confirmed by researchers investigating ultradian rhythms.[1] These are biological rhythms occurring more than once per day, the most fundamental ultradian rhythm being the basic rest and activity cycle.

It was conclusively shown, for instance, that there is an alternating nostril dominance, which means that the breath flows unevenly through the nostrils for periods of time. This suggests a still more basic vacillation in the processes of our nervous system.

These findings came as no surprise to *yogins*. For centuries they have known and used techniques for influencing the autonomous nervous system directly by way of controlled alternate breathing. This involves the careful regulation of the air flow through the nasal passages—a yogic science known as *svarodaya*.

The best known technique of alternate breathing is called *nadi-shodhana* or "cleansing the channels." This is executed by inhaling through one nostril and, after a spell of breath retention, exhaling through the other nostril. Often this practice is combined with varyingly complex visualizations.

Another technique of alternate breathing is called *surya-bheda-pranayama* or "breath control by means of piercing the sun," that is, activating the solar current of life-energy. This is done by inhaling through the right nostril and, after a period of breath retention (*kumbhaka*), exhaling through the left. This exercise, when repeated often enough, is said to clear the head and to cure diseases arising from an imbalance of the air element.

To return to our larger historical consideration: The adepts of *hatha-yoga* understood their teachings as a potent antidote to the Dark Age, the *kali-yuga*, which is thought to have commenced with the death of the God-man Krishna. The idea of world ages became popular in India around the turn of the first millennium A.D. and was closely associated with the emergence of Tantrism, which was promoted as a new spirituality particularly suited for "modern" humanity. According to native computations the *kali-yuga* will last until the year 428,898 A.D.!

Best described as a comprehensive cultural style analogous to the European Renaissance, Tantrism exerted a powerful influence on the Hindu, Buddhist, and also Jaina traditions. It espoused a down-to-earth, practical orientation centering on the "female energy" (*shakti*) as a psychic and cosmic principle. Religious and esoteric rituals figured prominently in this approach, because the Tantric masters deemed that most spiritual aspirants in the *kali-yuga* lacked the necessary discriminative intelligence (*buddhi*) and moral stamina for the higher contemplative practices. Ritual, which is always a bodily procedure, was considered the most appropriate means of focusing consciousness. A crucial aspect of this ritualism was the awakening of the "Goddess power," or "serpent power," in the body.

Neither Indian puritanism nor Western sensationalism does justice to the sublime esoteric teachings of Tantrism, which were crucial to the development of Indian civilization because they offered a new appraisal of human embodiment and physical reality. For centuries the Indian saints and sages, emphasizing the "otherworldliness" of ultimate Reality, had denied themselves every human pleasure. They lived on a starvation diet, suppressed the sexual impulse, and dwelled in isolated caves and impenetrable forests, as far removed from the temptations of ordinary human life as possible.

The adepts of Tantrism turned all this around. They stopped looking at bodily existence as being in conflict with the highest spiritual reality. They saw it rather as a manifestation, a delightful play, of the all-pervading One Being. The Tantric masters treasured the human body as a temple of ultimate Reality and as an exceedingly valuable instrument for the realization of the enlightened condition.

This positive orientation gave rise to schools of *kaya-sadhana*, or "body cultivation," which worked with the various subtle energy bodies as well as the physical body. By mastering the life-force of the body, the Tantric adepts sought to bring about changes on the levels of energy and consciousness. This mastery was attempted primarily through breath control (*pranayama*) and the application of different bodily "locks" (*bandha*) and "seals" (*mudra*) that have a particularly strong effect on the body's hormonal system. But the key to "body cultivation" was always the mind—the disciplining of attention through concentration and meditation.

The Tantric ideal was to create an "adamantine body" (*vajra-deha*)—a body that could withstand the ordeal of higher spiritual practice. Spiritual life is a matter of intensifying one's awareness. During the initial stages of practice, as the practitioners of Yoga become conscious of hitherto unconscious patterns, they inevitably find themselves engaged in an inner struggle with their tendencies—a struggle that can easily weaken the body. *Kaya-sadhana* was invented to prevent such weakening. The Tantric practitioners wanted to steel the body for the high-energy event of enlightenment, and so they developed *kaya-sadhana*, which gradually evolved into *hatha-yoga*, with its numerous postures, locks, seals, and purificatory techniques.

Goraksha—whoever he may have been—is universally acknowledged as the founder of this form of Yoga. Legend also remembers him as a great miracle-worker who is said to have flown through the sky, shifted shapes, vanished into thin air, read people's innermost thoughts, conversed with nonhuman creatures, healed the sick, and even raised the dead.

Some of the many scriptures attributed to Goraksha still exist in manuscript form. Most later works draw from these scriptures—though probably Goraksha himself never committed a word to paper, but let his pupils and their pupils do all the writing.

Goraksha (in Hindi, Gorakh or Gorakhnath) is also celebrated as the founder of an order that boasts numerous members even today. Variously known as Gorakhnathis, Darshanis (from the large earrings they wear) or Kanpathas (lit., "split-eared"), his followers are mostly ascetics, though there are householders among them, and even a few practitioners of Tantric sexual rites. All of them worship the Divine in the form of Shiva, and all are part of an initiatory lineage.

The majority of Gorakhnathis today are sadly lacking in the lofty spirit of Goraksha's original teaching. In fact, only a few of his many thousands of followers seem to have any real knowledge of their tradition. Already in the fifteenth century, the poet Kabir criticized them for failing to understand the true purpose of Yoga. "Whose loss is it if they do not apply the philosopher's stone that Gorakhnath possessed?" he lamented in his *Bijak*.

Nevertheless, Goraksha's followers also included many great spiritual heroes, several kings, and a few poet laureates who upheld his high ideals. The second part of this essay will focus on their contribution to this history of *hatha-yoga*.

§

An all-time favorite of *hatha-yoga* practitioners, both in India and in the West, is the *Hatha-Yoga-Pradipika*. Written by Svatmarama, who probably lived in the fifteenth century, this work shows *hatha-yoga* in a highly developed form. In the opening verses, Svatmarama mentions a long list of *hatha-yoga* teachers starting with Lord Shiva himself. [2]

Most of these names are completely obscure, and they may have been no more than faint memories even in Svatmarama's time. But a few of them—like Caurangi and Allama Prabhudeva—have scriptures and stories associated with them.

Caurangi, for instance, is remembered as a disciple of Matsyendra, who also initiated Goraksha into the secrets of Yoga. Prince Caurangi's story is told in the Bengali drama *Full Moon*. Apparently his stepmother had his hands and feet cut off before having him abandoned in a forest. Matsyendra found him, saved his life, and adopted him as a pupil. After twelve years of intense practice, Caurangi grew back his limbs.

Allama Prabhudeva, who died in 1196 A.D., is said, according to a South Indian tradition, to have met Goraksha under some unusual circumstances. The story goes that Goraksha demonstrated to

Allama how he, Goraksha, had become invulnerable to any weapon. Allama then asked Goraksha to strike him with a sword. To Goraksha's amazement, the sword passed through Allama's body as if it were made of space. Allama explained that, when the illusion of having a body is canceled through Self-realization, the "frozen shadow" (i.e., the body) is also eliminated. According to a more credible account, Allama was the head of a remarkable fellowship of more than three hundred Self-realized practitioners, including sixty women.

As these stories demonstrate, psychic powers are an integral part of the history of Yoga. Even Patanjali dedicates an entire chapter to them, and Goraksha in particular is frequently depicted performing extraordinary magical feats.

If we want to understand the connection between Yoga and magic, however, we must set aside our materialistic, scientific framework and merely enjoy on their own terms the many splendid stories of men and women who have devoted their whole lives to discovering the secrets of the body and the mind.

As we have seen, nothing definite is known about Goraksha, the reputed founder of *hatha-yoga*. As with Jesus of Nazareth or Gautama the Buddha, we are largely dependent for our information on questionable stories and traditions, some of which are blatantly wrong, others largely legendary. What is certain, however, is that Goraksha was a remarkable spiritual teacher who vitalized the yogic tradition. His influence was kept alive throughout India by his numerous disciples, among the most renowned of whom were Bhartrihari and Gopicandra.

Bhartrihari abdicated the throne of the kingdom of Ujjain to become a *yogin* and went on to head one of the thirteen principal subsects of the religious order founded by Goraksha. Bhartrihari was apparently initiated by the famous adept Jalandhari, a disciple of Matsyendra, but is said to have acknowledged Goraksha as his *guru*.

The thirteenth-century drama by Harihara called *Bhartrihari's Indifference* relates the story of King Bhartrihari's renunciation. Wanting to test his wife's faithfulness, Bhartrihari sent her a false report of his death. In keeping with ancient custom, she promptly threw herself on the funeral pyre.

Bhartrihari was disconsolate at his wife's untimely death. When he heard that Goraksha might be able to relieve him of his grief, he invited the master to the palace. Taking in the king's situation at once, Goraksha immediately broke his begging bowl and started to weep bitterly over it. This was a profound lesson for Bhartrihari, who saw the parallel between the lovely bowl of clay and his wife's body. Vowing to renounce the world, he accepted Goraksha as his teacher. Goraksha restored the queen to life, but Bhartrihari remained firm in his resolution to live as an ascetic.

Another famous king whose name is frequently associated with Goraksha's is Gopicandra, who lived in the eleventh century. His story is told in the *Song of Manikcandra,* which is popular to this day throughout the northeast of India. According to this ballad, Gopicandra's mother was a pupil of Goraksha. When Goraksha realized that Gopicandra was destined to live a short life, he insisted that the young man abdicate the throne and become a *yogin.* Goraksha further instructed that he should accept as his *guru* a sweeper named Hadi.

Apart from resenting the idea of having a lowly sweeper for his teacher, Gopicandra suspected that Goraksha and his mother might be conspiring against him. So he put his mother to the test. She was made to walk on fire, given poison to swallow, and was submerged in water. But she survived all ordeals by invoking the name of her *guru.* At last Gopicandra was convinced that her demand for his abdication was free of ulterior motives, and he humbly asked Hadi to accept him as his student. His life as a *yogin* was filled with untold hardships.

Hadi is better known as Matsyendra's disciple Jalandhari, who is thought to have been the inventor of the classical "lock" bearing his name, in which the chin is pressed down on the chest to prevent the breath, or life-force, from escaping.

Whether true or not, such stories show that Goraksha's influence was not confined to the poor and illiterate. His teaching had appeal on all levels of society.

Indeed, one of India's greatest poets, Saint Jnanadeva (thirteenth century), traces his spiritual lineage back to Goraksha. Jnanadeva was initiated by his elder brother Nivritti, who was a pupil of Gahini. And Gahini was a direct disciple of Goraksha.

Jnanadeva was a spiritual and poetic genius. He wrote a celebrated Marathi verse commentary on the *Bhagavad-Gita* at the age of fifteen, and at his own request had himself buried alive in a vault six years later. Immersing himself in the ecstatic state (*samadhi*), he abandoned his body and never regained ordinary consciousness. Three centuries later his tomb (which has a strong spiritual presence to this day) caved in. Asked to inspect the remains, Saint Ekanatha reported that the body was still preserved, apparently through Jnanadeva's yogic powers.

Jnanadeva's works indicate that he was familiar with the great secret of Goraksha's Yoga—the "serpent power," or *kundalini-shakti,* the universal "deathless" energy. The *kundalini* is the power aspect of ultimate Reality, which is conceived as unqualified existence (*sat*), pure awareness (*cit*), and unsurpassable bliss (*ananda*).

The *kundalini* makes all life possible. It is at the root of all human activity and experience. But it is also the force that, when used with wisdom, can lead a person beyond all manifest worlds. It is extolled in the *hatha-yoga* scriptures as the hidden means to the conquest of death. In the words of the anonymous author of the *Yoga-Shikha-Upanishad* (VI. 55):

> For the *yogins,* the *kundalini-shakti* is conducive to liberation, but for fools it leads to bondage. He who knows that power is a knower of Yoga.

According to the esoteric philosophy of *hatha-yoga,* the human body is a miniature version of the universe. The scriptures speak of seven major structures (called *cakra*) that correspond to levels of cosmic existence. The universal energy, or *kundalini,* can be tapped in any of these seven structures or centers.

In *hatha-yoga,* the *kundalini* is most frequently contacted in the lowest center, located at the base of the spine. From there it is conducted upward to the top center at the crown of the head, the so-called thousand-petaled lotus. The ascent of the *kundalini* through the various centers is associated with all kinds of psychophysical changes in the body. These have been vividly described by the late Pandit Gopi Krishna, who enjoyed (and suffered) a spontaneous awakening of the *kundalini.* Gopi Krishna writes:

Suddenly, with a roar like that of a waterfall, I felt a stream of liquid light entering my brain through the spinal cord. . . . The illumination grew brighter and brighter, the roaring louder, I experienced a rocking sensation and then felt myself slipping out of my body, entirely enveloped in a halo of light.[3]

Gopi Krishna's experience was utterly blissful. But, like all experiences, it was impermanent. It did, however, change his body chemistry. He continued to perceive the world differently and was able to enter into that blissful state more readily. But for a very long time it also caused him unbelievable pain and torment. As he remembers:

I sometimes gagged my mouth to keep from crying and fled from the solitude of my room to the crowded street to prevent myself from doing some desperate act.[4]

Nevertheless, Gopi Krishna maintained that the "awakening of *kundalini* is the greatest enterprise and the most wonderful achievement of man."[5] He learned to contain the mysterious power that resides in the body. But containment is not mastery. Gopi Krishna's saintly life and numerous books notwithstanding, it seems unlikely that he was a full-fledged *kundalini-yogin.*

When the serpent power reaches the topmost center, the practitioners of this Yoga literally "blow their mind." They enter the ecstatic condition where they realize the flawless unity of all things. This is an indescribably blissful state in which self-consciousness is temporarily suspended. Unless the *kundalini* returns to the lower centers, the body dies after a period of time.

Because this experience is so overwhelming, it can easily traumatize the unprepared body-mind. Hence the masters of *hatha-yoga* have designed numerous purificatory techniques that help prepare the nervous system for the onslaught of the aroused *kundalini.*

The earliest *hatha-yoga* scriptures, like the *Siddha-Siddhanta-Paddhati* or *the Kaula-Jnana-Nirnaya*, do not mention any specific purificatory practice. But we must assume that such practices existed and were taught in secret. Possibly they comprised mostly breathing techniques and dietary rules that were intended to strengthen and stabilize the nervous system.

Later many other techniques were added to the yogic repertoire. We can get a glimpse of the evolution of these practices when we study the *Hatha-Yoga-Pradipika* (c. fifteenth century) and the *Gheranda-Samhita* (c. seventeenth century), which list and summarize more than twenty preparatory practices. Some of these are even recommended for curing specific ailments.

There even exists an eighteenth-century work, the *Sat-Karma-Samgraha*, which reads like a manual of yogic therapy. Traditional *hatha-yoga* is a dangerous tool, as many scriptures warn. In the course of one's practice, one may encounter all kinds of obstructions, and these in turn may trigger a dormant illness. Also, inattention or faulty practice can have undesirable side-effects, especially in the advanced stages of practice. The *Sat-Karma-Samgraha* ("Collection of Right Actions") is full of remedial measures.

Hatha-yogins treat the body as a laboratory. They do not desire a merely pleasant meditation while being abstracted from the body. On the contrary, they aspire to realize the blissfulness of the ultimate Reality in the context of the body. This is the spirit of Tantrism, where enlightenment or Self-realization is not an otherworldly experience. It is here and now, and therefore must include (and ultimately transform) the body.

There is no question that *hatha-yoga* evolved in close association with Ayurveda ("life science"), the native Indian medical tradition. Ayurveda and Yoga have many concepts and techniques in common. Some of the cleansing practices, in particular, appear to have derived directly from age-old medical lore.

Like the purificatory techniques, so did posture (*asana*), gesture (*mudra*), breath control (*pranayama*), concentration (*dharana*), and meditation (*dhyana*) evolve over the centuries, as *yogins* paid increasing attention to maintaining the body in optimal health. This trend is captured in the *Gheranda-Samhita* (I.2), which speaks of *hatha-yoga* as the "Yoga of the pot." The "pot" (*gatha*) is the body, which is like earthenware; in order to harden it, the text states, one must bake it in the fire of Yoga.

The development of the physical dimension of *hatha-yoga* became so exaggerated that nowadays many Indian and Western practitioners know little about its spiritual origins and purposes.

But divorced from its spiritual orientation, *hatha-yoga* is no more than calisthenics. It may help one to become more supple or to stay fit. But only when it is practiced with a spiritual intention can its secrets be unlocked.

To be sure, the goal of traditional *hatha-yoga* is not health but perfect well-being, which is founded on Self-realization. *Hatha-yoga* is meant not merely to cure illnesses but to unburden its practitioner from all suffering. And that is accomplished by dispelling the illusion that one is a separate being and by discovering the authentic Being, which is eternal, supraconscious, and blissful.

NOTES

1. See S. Anderson and G. Feuerstein, "Ultradian Rhythms in Science and Spiritual Practice," *Magical Blend*, no. 30 (January–April 1991), pp. 40–43.

2. Many works on Yoga are composed in verse. The meter is generally very simple and pleasant to the ear so that the verses can be readily memorized.

3. Gopi Krishna, *Kundalini: The Evolutionary Energy in Man* (London: Robinson & Watkins, 1971), pp. 12–13.

4. *Ibid.*, p. 51.

5. *Ibid.*, p. 243.

13

THE EVOLUTION OF POSTURE (ASANA)

At the heart of all forms of Yoga is the practice of meditation (*dhyana*), the stilling of the mind and the transcendence of ordinary consciousness. Even the Yoga of self-transcending action (*karma-yoga*), the most outgoing of yogic approaches, calls for what can be described as a meditative disposition in life. To meditate, however, one must first establish bodily equanimity.

Hence, the classical eightfold path taught by Patanjali in the *Yoga-Sutra* gives considerable weight to bodily posture (*asana*). In aphorisms II.46–48, Patanjali states:

> The posture [should be] stable and comfortable. [It is accompanied] by the relaxation of tension and [one's] coinciding with the infinite [consciousness-space]. Thence [comes] unassailability by the pairs-of-opposites.

This quite literal rendering of the aphorisms helps us get closer to Patanjali's original meaning.[1] What he is telling us in the first sentence is simply good common sense: We cannot have our arms and legs flailing about while we are trying to meditate. True, certain spiritual traditions, such as Hinayana Buddhism and Sufism, know of meditation exercises that are performed while moving about, but these practices generally involve intense self-observation, or witnessing, and have a great stillness and even elegance about them.

At any rate, Patanjali had something else in mind. For him, meditation is self-observation that is meant to lead to ecstatic self-transcendence in the state of *samadhi*. Since this elevated yogic state presupposes intense concentration and a loss of bodily awareness, it is easy to see why one should be seated in a stable, comfortable posture.

A successful posture implies, as Patanjali puts it, the release or relaxation of tension in which the bodily energies begin to flow freely. This relaxation is accompanied by a new sense of bodily existence. One feels as if one had expanded beyond one's skin, and the body is experienced as an unbounded field of energy. This is presumably what Patanjali had in mind when he speaks of "coinciding with the infinite (*ananta*)," meaning the infinite inner space of consciousness.

The more profound one's relaxation, the more successful one's posture. Patanjali even gives us an objective measure for determining the depth of our relaxation and *asana* practice, stating that successful practice leads to a state in which we become insensitive to what he calls the "pairs-of-opposites" (*dvandva*). These are such opposite sensations as heat and cold, humidity and aridity, pain and pleasure. In other words, *asana* contains an element of sensory withdrawal (*pratyahara*).

When the body is perfectly relaxed, a pin prick and, at a more advanced stage, even the dentist's drill fail to disturb our inner equilibrium. Body and mind cannot be separated other than in the abstract, and posture is, if truly practiced, a demanding exercise involving both body and consciousness.

Long before Patanjali codified the yogic practices and ideas prevalent in his time, the mystics and ascetics of the Indian subcontinent had recognized the importance of a stable posture for the practice of sensory inhibition (*pratyahara*), concentration (*dharana*), and meditation (*dhyana*).

Thus the ancient *Atharva-Veda*, which is part of the sacred canon of Hinduism, mentions wandering mystics, the Vratyas, who were forerunners of the *yogins* of later times. These Vratyas, who lived some three thousand years ago, used music, song, and dance in their mystical rituals. Their religious paraphernalia included a seat (called *asandi*), around which was woven a detailed metaphysical symbolism. The use of this seat would seem to show that the Vratyas had recognized the important role played by a steady posture in the spiritual task of internalizing consciousness.

The Vratyas also speculated extensively about the nature of the breath, or life-force (*prana*), and invented breathing exercises that, in the course of time, evolved into the typical yogic techniques of breath control (*pranayama*).

The Buddhist scriptures describe Gautama the Buddha's great penance before his spontaneous enlightenment under a fig tree. They portray him as having wrestled with himself in meditation until sweat poured from his whole body. At the time, he was seated cross-legged in the so-called *paryanka* seat, or squatting position.

The Buddha's austerities lasted six years, during much of which time he sat in perfect stillness, fiercely focusing his mind. His "sitting" was extraordinary but not atypical. He had undoubtedly learned it during his discipleship with different Yoga masters, two of whom are even mentioned by name in the Buddhist canonical literature.

In the *Bhagavad-Gita* (VI.11–14), the earliest and most popular Yoga scripture, the God-man Krishna instructs his pupil Arjuna thus:

> Setting up a steady seat for himself in a pure place, neither too high nor too low, with a cloth, deer-skin, or grass upon it—there making the mind one-pointed, restraining the activity of mind and senses, he should, seated on the seat, yoke himself in Yoga for the purification of the self. Equable, keeping trunk, head, and neck motionless and steady, gazing at the tip of the nose, without looking round about him, with tranquil self and devoid of fear, steadfast in the vow of celibacy, controlling the mind, his thoughts on Me, yoked—he should sit intent on Me.

Here, as in the early *Upanishads*, it is still the physical seat that is called *asana*. But we are also given a clear description of the yogic meditation posture to which that Sanskrit term came later to be applied. The *Bhagavad-Gita* belongs to the third or perhaps fourth century B.C. Yoga had barely been systematized at that time. A century or two later, the anonymous author of the *Maitrayaniya-Upanishad* made a first attempt at systematizing the yogic path, but he still does not mention posture as a separate "limb."

That innovation first appears in the *Yoga-Sutra*, though even here we find an echo of the earlier meaning of the word *asana*. "Posture" is, of course, a generic term, and from ancient times *yogins* had undoubtedly used different kinds of postures to immobilize the body for meditation.

In the *Yoga-Bhashya* ("Discourses on Yoga"), the oldest extant commentary on Patanjali's aphorisms, several such postures are mentioned by name: "lotus posture" (*padma-asana*), "hero posture" (*vira-asana*), "auspicious posture" (*bhadra-asana*), "well- being posture" (*svastika-asana*), "staff posture" (*danda-asana*), and posture "with support" (*sa-upashraya*). The anonymous author of the *Bhashya*, who is traditionally identified as Vyasa, composer of a great national epic, mentions several others: "couch" (*paryanka*), "curlew seat" (*kraunca-nishadana*), "elephant seat" (*hasti-nishadana*), "camel seat" (*ushtra-nishadana*), and "even arrangement" (*sama-samsthana*).

These names are fascinating, and some of the poses, like the lotus and the hero, are well known even today. Others we can identify from modern manuals or guess at from their names. But a good many would be a complete enigma without the explanations of later Sanskrit commentators. Thus Vacaspati Mishra, a great ninth-century scholar who also wrote a commentary on Patanjali's work, supplies some valuable though sketchy descriptions.

The auspicious posture, according to Vacaspati, is performed by bringing the soles of the feet together close to the genitals. Then the hands are placed over the feet "in the shape of a tortoise." The *svastika* posture is described in terms suggesting that it resembles the lotus posture. The staff posture is executed by extending the legs with the feet next to each other. The posture "with support" is so called because it involves the use of a "yogic table" (*yoga-pattaka*).

According to Vacaspati, the "couch" is performed by lying down with the arms cradling the knees. In other writings, this posture is described as a squatting pose. The "even arrangement" is practiced with the feet close together and, presumably, sitting on one's heels. Vacaspati laconically observes that the animal "seats" may be understood by observing animals themselves.

It is interesting to note that at the time of Vyasa, in the fifth century, a distinction was made between *asanas* and *nishadanas*, the latter apparently being postures that imitated animals. The word *nishadana* ("sitting down") is almost synonymous with the word *upanishad* ("sitting down close to"), which refers to esoteric teachings originally handed down from teacher to pupil by word of mouth. During these oral transmissions, the pupil would sit close to the teacher, presumably in one or another yogic posture.

Four advanced yogic postures (asana) *performed by Theos Bernard, one of the early exponents of* hatha-yoga *in the West.*

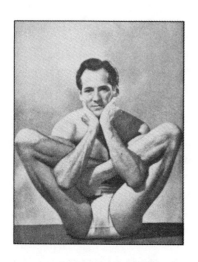

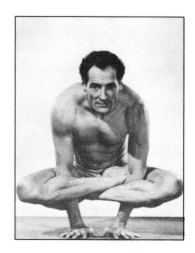

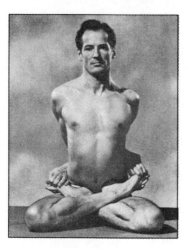

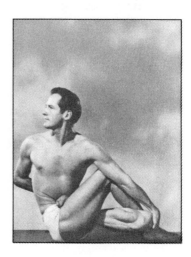

The lotus posture—the *asana* frequently associated with meditation—is the most stable of the sitting poses, and stability was undoubtedly the principal objective of many of the other postures as well. Sitting cross-legged on the ground came (and still comes) naturally to the Indians. Nonetheless, the practice of folding one leg over the other was an important innovation.

Practitioners of yogic *asanas* must have discovered quite early an interesting fact that can easily be verified today by anyone sensitive to it: By assuming a yogic posture, one automatically changes the flow of life-energy in the body, which manifests in subtle alterations of one's mood or body awareness. These changes are to some degree even measurable by clinical means.[2]

In her pioneering work *Where the Spirits Ride the Wind*, Felicitas D. Goodman has described different postures used in archaic Shamanism to bring about ecstatic states.[3] Her research, however, has not been purely historical or ethnographic. She and her students also experimented with these postures, achieving astonishing results.

The discovery that posture has a significant effect on our inner world must have prompted the *yogins* to experiment with different postures and their effect on the body and consciousness. Living close to Nature, they looked to the animal kingdom for inspiration and so created a variety of postures with animal names.

For a very long time, their chief purpose in using *asanas* must have been to enhance meditation practice. Yet certainly these Yoga practitioners could not have helped but notice the effects their *asanas* had on the physical body and its general well-being. That we have no records for these therapeutic discoveries until much later does not mean that they were not made in those early days. The literature of the native medical system, which is also quite ancient, makes it clear that Yoga was one of the major sources of inspiration for the naturopathic doctors of India.

Not until the advent of Tantrism, however, toward the end of the first post-Christian millennium, could the therapeutic value of the Yoga postures and other exercises (notably breath control) come to the fore. Tantrism was a new cultural style that affected the whole of Indian civilization, introducing a more down-to-earth religious attitude that included a new orientation toward bodily existence, sexuality, and (to some extent) the female gender. As explained in the preceding essay, the "Tantric revolution" gave rise to an entirely new type of Yoga—*hatha-yoga.*

The masters of this renaissance Yoga still taught the supreme goal of enlightenment and the royal road of meditation. But they adopted a different approach, paying considerable attention to preparing the body for the sacred ordeal of the higher phases of Yoga. They greatly elaborated the postures and breathing techniques and invented a whole battery of cleansing practices.

The *Goraksha-Samhita* ("Goraksha's Collection"), belonging perhaps to the twelfth or thirteenth century, is one of the first works to mention three major "locks" (*bandha*), which can be considered a type of posture. These "locks" are respectively applied to the anus, the abdomen, and the throat in conjunction with breath retention. Today advanced *hatha-yoga* practice is unthinkable without these innovative techniques.

Breath control is crucial since it is through controlled breathing (or breath retention) that the "serpent power," the *kundalini*, is awakened and manipulated. This mysterious life-force, which is fundamental to all *hatha-yoga* and Tantric practice, is considered the agency by which a person is either bound and deluded or liberated and enlightened.

Not surprisingly, the earliest *hatha-yoga* scriptures already emphasized breathing techniques, often in combination with *mantra* recitation. Over the centuries this aspect was developed into a great art, and later texts describe a variety of techniques for regulating the breath. Some works, like the *Svara-Cintamani* and the *Shiva-Svarodaya,* explain how the breath can be used for diagnostic and divinatory purposes. Here Yoga wisdom and medical practice overlap. Often specific postures are prescribed for certain breathing exercises.

We can only marvel at the ingenuity and inventiveness of the Indian *yogins* and their acute observations and experimental attitude. This is particularly apparent in the case of the postures. The *Gheranda-Samhita* ("Gheranda's Collection"), a late-seventeenth-century text that is still very popular among modern *yogins*, mentions thirty-two postures and twenty-five "gestures" (*mudra*), in addition to twenty-one preparatory practices.

This medieval Sanskrit work represents a major development.

Not only did the postures grow in number, they also acquired a new function. Many could not possibly be used for prolonged meditation. Instead, they have a different purpose, which is repeatedly pointed out in the various descriptions. "Such-and-such a posture," we are constantly being told, "cures such-and-such a disease"—or even all ailments.

Thus there are two basic kinds of posture: those that primarily serve the meditative process and those that are chiefly intended to purify and balance the body. Of course, there is some overlap: Meditative *asanas* such as the lotus posture are also said to have curative value, and therapeutic *asanas* like the headstand (*shirsha-asana*) can be used for meditation as well. Theos Bernard, the first Western scholar to submit to a classical training in *hatha-yoga*, learned to meditate in the headstand for an hour or more.

Significantly, the term *shirsha-asana* is a relatively recent coinage. In the *Gheranda-Samhita* and other traditional manuals, the practice is listed not among the postures but among the "gestures" (*mudra*). The reason for this is that the headstand, properly executed, is an incredibly potent exercise with a powerful impact on the hormonal system. Although all yogic practices are designed to bring about changes in body chemistry (and hence in consciousness), the *mudras* are singled out for their immense effectiveness.

The meaning of the word *mudra*, literally "seal," hints at the fact that in the techniques the so-called life-current (*prana*) is "sealed" in the body and thus contained so that it can be mobilized for the practice of concentration and meditation.

Historically, the principal *mudras* are older than the therapeutic *asanas*. The former were invented or discovered in experimenting with breath control and mental concentration. The latter are "technological" refinements that belong to a later age, perhaps the fourteenth or fifteenth century, and came to be associated with what in the *Gheranda-Samhita* is called *ghatastha-yoga*, the "Yoga of the pot." The "pot" refers to the human body, and the philosophy behind this phrase is given in the opening section (verse 8) of that manual:

> The "pot" invariably wears away like an unbaked earthen jar immersed in water. [Therefore] one should cultivate the "pot's" perfection by burning it in the fire of Yoga.

The host of postures and cleansing practices we encounter in the late classical and modern manuals of *hatha-yoga* are designed to "bake" the body or, as we would say, steel it. In the *Gheranda-Sambita* (I.10–11) we read:

> Purification [of the body is accomplished] by means of the six preparatory acts; strengthening, by means of the postures; steadiness, by means of the "gestures"; tranquillity, by means of sense-withdrawal; lightness, by means of breath control; [initial] perception of the self, by means of meditation; and undiminished freedom is undoubtedly [accomplished] by means of ecstasy (*samadhi*).

Of course, the postures do more than strengthen the body, as is clear from the claims made in the scriptures. And in contemporary Yoga practice, both East and West, they are often given precedence over all other limbs of Yoga. But Yoga is a holistic system in which every aspect is in balance with every other aspect. At the center of it all is the spiritual aspiration toward enlightenment, or freedom from conditioning—from our egoic personality. In other words, self-transcendence is the supreme value, not merely physical well-being or superior functioning.

The postures are only one branch of the large tree of Yoga. Although they can be health-building when practiced on their own, their real benefits are best enjoyed when they are cultivated as an integral part of the total way of life that is *hatha-yoga*.

NOTES

1. For a complete translation, see G. Feuerstein, *The Yoga-Sutra* (Rochester, VT: Inner Traditions, 1989).

2. See, e.g., the study by the Canadian psychologist V.F. Emerson, "Can Belief Systems Influence Behavior? Some Implications of Research on Meditation," *Newsletter Review*, the R.M. Bucke Memorial Society, vol. 5 (1972), pp. 20–32.

3. See F.D. Goodman, *Where the Spirits Ride the Wind: Trance Journeys and Other Ecstatic Experiences* (Bloomington: Indiana University Press, 1990).

14

THE SERPENT POWER (KUNDALINI-SHAKTI) AND THE SPIRITUAL LIFE: IN DIALOGUE WITH LEE SANNELLA, M.D.

Lee Sannella is a psychiatrist and an ophthalmologist. His book *The Kundalini Experience* was first published in 1976 and has since been praised as a classic in the literature on the interface between psychiatry and mysticism. Dr. Sannella is also a co-founder of the Kundalini Clinic in Oakland, California, which over the years has helped numerous "victims" of spontaneous *kundalini* awakenings.

GF: Your book *The Kundalini Experience* has brought a new understanding to a very intriguing phenomenon—the *kundalini-shakti*, or "serpent power." This power is traditionally thought to underlie all psychic and spiritual processes, even the biological processes of the body. I want to ask you a number of questions about this. But first, how did you, a medical doctor and psychiatrist, become interested in such a relatively obscure phenomenon?

LS: It all started with a trip to the Far East back in, I think, 1973 or 1974. I went to Japan with my friend the late Itzhak Bentov to do some research in Hiroshi Motoyama's laboratory. We wanted to duplicate the experiments Bentov had conducted with his accelerometer measuring the body's micromotion. Motoyama's lab had fairly sophisticated equipment, which allowed more accurate readings—particularly bilateral tracings of the head. Bentov was one of the few people able to induce what is called the resonance state at will. He was to be our guinea pig. He would get into resonance, and then we took our various measurements. To our amazement, we discovered that the left side of Bentov's head showed greater amplitude than the right—a sign of *kundalini* activity.

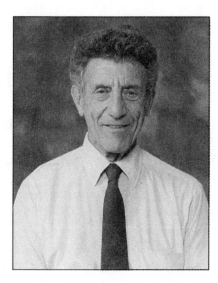

Lee Sannella

As I understand it, on the basis of Bentov's model, the *kundalini* awakening is the product of a resonance state, which is attained either spontaneously or through prolonged spiritual discipline such as meditation. Bentov showed that the heart-aorta system produces an oscillation in the body, including the skull, of a frequency of about 7 Hz. (i.e., 7 cycles per second). The oscillation in the skull in turn produces acoustical plane waves reverberating through the brain at kilohertz frequencies. The standing waves in the skull in turn generate a pulsating magnetic field that, Bentov speculated, interacts with the electro-magnetic fields in the environment. Specifically, during deep meditation the phenomenon of "rhythm entrainment" occurs, whereby the meditator goes into sine-wave oscillation at approximately 7 Hz., which tends to lock him (or her) into the frequency of the planetary atmosphere. Bentov's physiological model explains, among other things, why the *kundalini* effect occasionally occurs in nonmeditators, through purely mechanical stimulation such as a loud, persistent sound.

Now, at the time of our trip, Bentov was undergoing what I later understood to have been full-fledged *kundalini* activity. He had visionary experiences and involuntary bodily movements called *kriyas* (lit., "activities") in Yoga, and these manifestations would become stronger whenever he sat down to meditate. Several times he woke up in the middle of the night complaining that *shakti* was having him in her grip. So, I was given a firsthand demonstration of the *kundalini* phenomenon.

Next I came across an article on the African !Kung bushmen that talked about their extensive experience of the *kundalini*. It intrigued me that this experience should be known outside India and China. I began to investigate the *kundalini* phenomenon more seriously. At that time I still had no intention of writing a book about it. Then Bentov made it very clear to me that he was primarily interested in the cosmological side of the *kundalini*, rather than its medical, cross-cultural, or psychological aspects. I didn't see anyone else around at the time who might have tackled those other areas, so I began to work on a manuscript that grew into *The Kundalini Experience*.

GF: In your book you bring a whole series of case histories of men and women who have undergone the *kundalini* experience. How did you collect those?

LS: Well, Bentov obviously was the first case. Then there was his wife, who also had an active *kundalini* from her meditation practice. While we were still in the Far East, we got to meet a number of other people who shared their experiences with us. Back in the States, I discovered that a good many of the people experiencing *kundalini* had awakened the serpent power through psychedelic drugs.

GF: What is your attitude about the use of such drugs?

LS: I think they are mostly misused. They should be used as a sacrament, including marijuana. If they are used sacramentally, which means in moderation and with the purpose of opening up our psychic dimension, they are in my mind legitimate. In those days, however, drugs were mainly used for what I consider to be the wrong reasons—for social and sexual reasons or purely for self-gratification.

GF: You experimented with drugs yourself.

LS: Yes, and I believe we used them reasonably. We took or administered psychedelic drugs in a pleasant, quiet, and protected environment, where the person was alone but with help close by in case it was needed—sometimes even with a clairvoyant standing by to give us a better reading of the subject's inner states. Our whole objective was to invite a state of transcendence in that person. We used to call it "dropping the body." I was also indirectly connected with a research group in Palo Alto, which explored psychotomimetic drugs more systematically than I and my friends did. For us it was more a matter of exploring ourselves.

GF: But you didn't do drugs only?

LS: That's right. I was also practicing Zen and other forms of spiritual discipline. One of the methods I got involved with was the meditation taught by Swami Muktananda. In fact, it was with several of Muktananda's students that I started the Kundalini Clinic in the Bay area. One of them was Gabriel Cousens, a medical doctor, teacher, and writer, whom I introduced to Swami Muktananda. Recently he authored the book *The Rainbow Diet.* However, the Kundalini Clinic is run today by Stuart Sovatsky, a psychotherapist.

GF: Wouldn't you say it is remarkable for a psychiatrist to become a student of an Indian *guru*?

LS: Oh, I had been going to various spiritual teachers since the mid-1950s. Somehow I have always been interested in the spiritual. At home I was given no religious training at all, but I remember being very fascinated whenever I had the opportunity to listen to Bible readings in school. Perhaps this is why I became a Quaker in 1948.

After my experiences with LSD and other hallucinogens, I seriously delved into the psychic dimension of life. I researched psychics, healers, poltergeist phenomena, and so on. I also studied seven years with a teacher of the Gurdjieff tradition. I experienced the Gurdjieff system—at least the way it was taught to me—as suppressive rather than liberating. So, I turned to Zen Buddhism next. I wasn't a talented meditator at all. I had to work hard at it. For four solid months

I sat on my tailbone for as many hours as I possibly could. During that period I went to four *seshins*, sitting 10–12 hours a day for between three to seven days. By the time of the last *seshin*, I was in considerable physical discomfort, but more than that, really upset, frustrated, and confused.

I complained to my teacher, and he just told me to go back to sitting. "What will your friends think of you?" he added. He knew where to get me. A few hours later, he interviewed me again and, to my surprise, passed me. I protested because I didn't feel any different. Nothing had happened. I told him he was just kidding me. Something happened the next day, however.

I went for another interview and was rather cantankerous. My teacher told me to sit down, saying I would be alright. I sat down, and suddenly my mind simply evaporated. My mind was gone. Then an answer to a puzzle that had been pestering me for years and years suddenly loomed in my awareness: *God is.* I was overjoyed, ecstatic. I felt a great love that removed all differences. I wanted to tell everyone that there was no point in being judgemental about anything, because everything was as it should be. This state lasted for about thirty minutes.

Two days later a similar state overtook me. I was on a bus at the time, riding to work. I "heard" the bus driver "talking" to the bus, and I "heard" the tires "talking" to the bus. Everything had become transparent to me. I worked in this state the entire day. Then it faded, never to return again. Not so far anyway.

GF: Maybe you were trying too hard to make it happen?

LS: Sure. [*Laughter*] It taught me that I can break through to the spiritual dimension, and it showed me the inner condition that is necessary for such a breakthrough.

GF: With Muktananda, transmission—what he called *shakti-pata*—played an important role. How did this manifest in your case?

LS: Oh, he undoubtedly worked very hard on me but I wasn't too sensitive to his transmission, or to psychic energies in general. Of course, you can imagine all sorts of things, but I am not one to make claims that I don't feel to be real. My receptivity has, however, changed somewhat over time.

GF: To get back to the *kundalini*: How do you explain your various psychic and spiritual experiences in terms of the *kundalini* phenomenon?

LS: That's a big question. I became interested in the *kundalini* because I felt and still feel that it is the master condition that gives rise to the great variety of psychic and spiritual states that can be experienced. My *satori* experience was a function of the *kundalini*. My visionary experiences were caused by the *kundalini*. And the *kundalini* underlies anyone's spiritual or psychic experiences. It is the universal trigger for all these experiences.

There are also all kinds of prodromata, or manifestations, that precede the full-blown *kundalini* awakening. For instance, I nowadays predictably experience during meditation, but also occasionally at other times, a pressure or feeling of energy in the area of the forehead, the third eye. That sensation is part of the *kundalini* syndrome. Others have more complex symptoms. I believe that when I manage to make a deeper and also more predictable psychic connection with my present teacher, I am likely to experience stronger manifestations of such psychic energies.

GF: In your book you suggest that the *kundalini* mechanism has the evolutionary purpose of helping us to transcend the body-mind, and yet you and others who write about the *kundalini* mention a whole range of strange or unusual physical symptoms associated with an awakening of the serpent power.

LS: Well, as I see it, the many physical manifestations of the *kundalini* don't cancel its spiritual purpose. On the contrary, it is through the refinement of the physical, as it is accomplished through the *kundalini* process, that transcendence of the body-mind is made possible. It is a process of bodily transmutation by which the Divine becomes transparent to us. The Divine abides beyond the *kundalini* just as it abides beyond the body-mind. We realize it, however, in and through the body.

GF: Some great adepts like Gautama the Buddha appear to have reached full enlightenment without ever mentioning the *kundalini*. Other enlightened adepts have waxed eloquent about the *kundalini* and its numerous manifestations in the body. How do you explain this historical fact? Did they experience different forms of enlighten-ment?

LS: No, I believe full enlightenment is the same everywhere. The differences in this case can be explained as a matter of physical and mental constitution. For instance, the !Kung bushmen think that more emotional people can enter more readily into the *kundalini* state, which they call *n/um.* This is also my experience.

More intellectual types don't tend to experience *kundalini* a-rousal in as dramatic a way as more sensate or affective types. So, on the way to enlightenment, all kinds of psychic or spiritual or even somatic phenomena can occur (or not occur), but in each and every case the entire spiritual process is governed by the *kundalini* mechanism.

I should add that not everyone understands enlightenment in the same way, which has led to a great deal of confusion. For instance, the Zen masters distinguish between fleeting *satoris* lasting a few seconds or minutes, and the condition of final enlightenment which is permanent. It is the permanent condition that I am talking about. The short, momentary states of enlightenment are wonderful and may hold great personal significance, but they are merely signs along the road . . .

GF: . . . Which means we mustn't get too fixated on them.

LS: Right. They are valid as a moment of enlightenment, but that's all.

GF: And having such transitory *satori* experiences doesn't really tell you much about the *being* of a person.

LS: Yes, I have known very skilled meditators who enjoyed frequent *satoris* but also suffered from all kinds of psychological conditions that could be qualified as pathological. On the other hand, even pathological conditions can have a positive spiritual value if we relate to them rightly, that is, if they help us embrace reality more adequately.

GF: Let me push you a little on this. Could one say that the physi-cal *kundalini* manifestations are pathological but have a positive function?

LS: You could put it that way. Some manifestations clearly are pathological in the broader sense of the term, insofar as they are deviations from the norm and because they are outside a person's conscious control. Also, if a person were to get completely obsessed with those manifestations without applying discrimination to them, we would obviously be dealing with a case of pathology. Such a person would be a *kundalini* victim.

Gopi Krishna's case, for instance, included many pathological aspects. But he succeeded in bringing the *kundalini* manifestations under control and in turning the awakened *kundalini* into a benign force in his life. Some of my clients have done the same.

Generally, pathological manifestations occur when the *kundalini* is awakened accidentally and when there is no guidance, or when such states are taboo in the larger culture. Then the mind begins to play tricks on the person. This is why the right context is so important, and why a teacher is necessary.

GF: Your particular contribution to the study of the *kundalini* mechanism was to show that the physical symptoms associated with it can be regarded separately. You coined the term *physio-kundalini* to describe this symptom pattern.

LS: Yes. You see, this is the aspect of the *kundalini* process that can be studied. It is accessible to the outside observer. The symptoms are often very dramatic and florid. Everything else that is happening on the psychic level is private and rather inaccessible. We can get self-reports about psychic states, of course, but these aren't always reliable or even intelligible; whereas tremors of the limbs, manifestations of heat in the body, and so on, can be observed and measured.

GF: Could it be that the more florid manifestations, or even all physical manifestations associated with the *kundalini* process, are due to psycho-energetic blockages in the body? In other words, they are not necessarily signs of spiritual merit.

LS: Yes, but it seems that people experiencing such phenomena also are more sensitive. So, the symptoms are not merely a negative sign. They also tell us something about the individual's psychic sensitivity. This is similar to schizophrenia where the person is not merely crazy but also hypersensitive to sensory input and so on. They are overwhelmed by the information coming from the environment.

GF: Now, someone might ask: If the *kundalini* is the primary evolutionary mechanism that moves us toward the Divine and if it seems to be accessible through the body, then shouldn't we try everything possible to trigger it? For instance, to put it graphically, would it not be reasonable to jolt the *kundalini* into action by repeated bumps to the coccyx, where the process tends to start?

LS: [*Laughter*] This is indeed the recommendation of some teachers and schools. It is not something I would recommend.

GF: What do you recommend for a person who is experiencing an accidental awakening of the *kundalini*?

LS: I would suggest that they look for a qualified teacher and adopt a course of spiritual disciplines and seriously adhere to them. I believe that the more disturbing side-effects of the *kundalini* process are much more amenable to regulation when one observes regular spiritual disciplines. But having a teacher is very important. I think that 99.9 percent of all people require a teacher, a guide. Very few can stay on the spiritual path on their own.

GF: What virtues should a spiritual aspirant cultivate?

LS: I feel that integrity is one of the most important qualities, which any respectable teacher calls for. In ordinary life, as you know, we have hardly any use for integrity, and most people don't even know what spiritual integrity and spiritual discipline stand for.

GF: What role does love play in spiritual life?

LS: As I see it, the Divine is goodness, beauty, truth, and love. Without love, nothing has any value. You can experience all kinds of inner states and have all kinds of psychic abilities, but if you don't know how to attune yourself to that love, how to love, they amount to nothing.

GF: Let me pop the big question now: Have you yourself ever experienced the *kundalini*?

LS: No. I have had strong flows of energy in the body, pressure, and heat, but none of the other symptoms that are associated with the *physio-kundalini.* Maybe with further practice I will undergo a full-fledged *kundalini* experience, but I doubt it. I am constitutionally not particularly suited for it.

GF: Why have you for so many years written and spoken about the *kundalini?* What good can it do us to have information about this phenomenon?

LS: The significance doesn't lie so much in the *kundalini* phenomenon as in the condition of enlightenment to which it ultimately leads. Our culture needs to hear about the possibility of realizing the Divine. We are stuck, and I believe that hearing this message is essential. Otherwise, I don't think anything will change, and change clearly needs to occur.

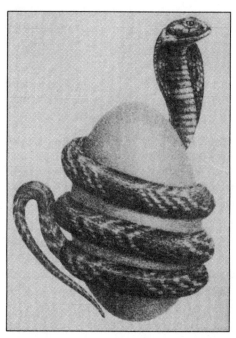

The image of the serpent coiled around an egg suggests the **kundalini** *in its macrocosmic aspect, with the egg representing the cosmos at large.*

15

TARAKA-YOGA: THE PATH OF LIGHT

The vast treasure-house of Indian esoteric knowledge has hardly been tapped as yet. What are a mere two hundred years of piecemeal scholarship compared to three millennia of experimentation and development? For this is the considerable space of time that Yoga has taken to reach its present shape. Considering the persistent stepmotherly treatment of Indian esoteric lore at the hand of Western orientalists, it is not really surprising that there are still innumerable gaps in our knowledge and understanding of Yoga. Many of its more obscure aspects have escaped the notice of the historians of religion. One of these gaps concerns the mysterious *taraka-yoga*.

The Sanskrit word *taraka* means "that which delivers" and in this particular school of Yoga the term stands for a definite set of yogic experiences. These are thought to conduct the *yogin* across the threshold of the world as we know it into the realm of the Unconditioned, the Real. Nothing is known about the history of this school except that it was probably established in the heyday of Tantrism at the beginning of the second millennium A.D. It is quite possible that at one time *taraka-yoga* attracted a large following from among the hundreds of thousands of spiritual seekers of medieval India.

Two Sanskrit texts setting forth this tradition have come down to our age, namely, the *Advaya-Taraka-Upanishad* and the *Mandala-Brahmana-Upanishad*. The former consists of nineteen verses, while the latter is a more elaborate version comprising ninety-one sections. Both scriptures belong to the medieval period, though their exact age is unknown.

Taraka-yoga is based on the nondualist philosophy of Advaita Vedanta. A fairly intricate system of thought formulated in its classical form by the renowned Shankara Acarya, who lived in the late eighth century A.D., Advaita Vedanta can be said to constitute the mainstream of contemporary Indian philosophy. Despite its considerable complexity, the principal axioms of this school can easily be grasped. In the *Viveka-Cudamani* ("Crest-Jewel of Discernment"), a popular work of edification, the doctrine is put in a nutshell thus:

> This entire universe, which through our spiritual blindness assumes manifold forms, is really nothing but *brahman* full free of any defects. (227)

> A pot, though a product of clay, is not anything different from it. For the pot is essentially the same as the clay. Why then call it a pot? It is a fictitious, constructed name merely. (228)

> Similarly, the whole world, being the effect of the real *brahman*, is nothing but that *brahman*. He who says it is something other than *brahman* babbles like one who is asleep. (230)

> Hence whatever is manifested as this world is the supreme *brahman* only, [which is] real, nondual, pure, of the essence of Awareness, taintless, tranquil, without beginning or end, inactive, of the nature of endless bliss. (237)

> That supreme *brahman* which transcends all speech is accessible to the eye of pure enlightenment. It is pure Awareness, the beginningless Reality. You are that *brahman*! Contemplate it yourself. (255)

The mystical experience of the singular Being, called *brahman* or *atman,* is so overpowering that the adepts are absolutely convinced that they have encountered something that is infinitely more real than anything related by the senses. They do not deny the myriad of forms in the universe. Their argument is rather that the senses do not give us a true picture of what there is. They firmly maintain that the mind of the unenlightened individual positively distorts reality by splitting it up into so many compartments. These compartments are the multiple entities located in the space-time world as we encounter it. In contrast, the single Being is an uninterrupted continuum where time stands still and the concept "space" is meaningless.

Since the world of multiplicity is the result of imperfect knowledge or spiritual blindness (*avidya*) that blocks out the knowledge of the single Being, it logically follows that this ultimate Real must also be our true nature.

It is the underlying purpose of any form of Yoga to eliminate all false identities that a person assumes in the course of a lifetime, and to bring the spiritual aspirant to his or her authentic identity, which is none other than the transcendental Ground or Self. When looked upon as the ultimate foundation of the manifold universe, this singular Reality is called *brahman,* whilst from a psychological viewpoint as the inmost essence of the person it is designated as *atman.* *Brahman* and *atman* signify one and the same all-pervasive Being.

The recovery of our true nature takes place in the act of enlightenment (*bodhi*) through the agency of Yoga. The process leading up to this supreme illumination is always the same: The mind is withdrawn from all external things and centered inward either with or without the help of a "prop," such as a potent sound (*mantra*) or a potent mental image (*yantra*), and so on.

In *taraka-yoga,* the switch by which the ordinary consciousness is converted into the continuous Awareness (*cit*) of the single Being is a series of exercises in which light phenomena play a decisive role. That inner light is produced by a technique known as *shambhavi-mudra* in Tantrism and *hatha-yoga.* Seated comfortably in the *siddha-asana* or any other posture, the *yogins* fix their sight on the cavern in the middle of the space between the eyebrows. The eyes can either be open or closed, the eyebrows may be slightly raised.

Whichever way it is executed, this practice always involves a new kind of looking by means of which the area of the forehead is brought into focus and somehow "energized." In terms of the esoteric physiology of *hatha-yoga* it implies the activation of the sixth center, the so-called *ajna-cakra.*

The light phenomena experienced in *taraka-yoga* do not derive from any external source such as the sun or other luminous objects. These lights are of a very special nature and are absolutely private occurrences. It is difficult to say precisely what they are. Neurophysiology and the psychology of altered states of consciousness are still in their infancy and do not have much to offer in the line of a sound explanation. At any rate it would be totally misleading to regard these experiences as due merely to the excitation of the optical nerves. They differ qualitatively from the kind of light flashes produced by, say, manual stimulation of the optical nerves.

Nor must these photisms be confused with hypnagogic images as experienced before sleep. The *taraka*-lights are extremely vivid and have a stunning quality of authenticity and reality. Whatever they may be in medical terms, to the practitioners of Yoga they represent signs of progress on the inward path. As practitioners succeed in emptying their mind of the sensory input and the images or word fragments bubbling up from the subconscious, their experience of radiant light becomes increasingly more intense and real.

According to the *Advaya-Taraka-Upanishad* there are three clearly discernible stages of achievement on this path of Yoga. These are referred to as the "three signs" (*tri-lakshya*). The first is known as the "inner sign" (*antar-lakshya*), the second as the "external sign" (*bahir-lakshya*), and the third as the "intermediate sign" (*madhya-lakshya*). These can be said to constitute different phases of *shambhavi-mudra*, the "gesture" or "seal" of Shambhu, Lord Shiva.

In keeping with Tantric imagery and its detailed esoteric "geography" of the human body, the *Advaya-Taraka-Upanishad* provides a concise description of the subtle energy centers and channels. According to this text, the axis of the body extending from the perineum to the crown of the head is a luminous channel in which is seated the mysterious force called *kundalini-shakti.*

This "serpent power" is described as being radiant like myriads of lightning-flashes. Even though resting dormant at the bottom of the central duct, the *kundalini* illuminates the entire channel known as the *sushumna-nadi.* This indescribable luminosity can be seen by *yogins* when they focus their inward eye on the "mental window" situated at the forehead. This locus is technically referred to as *lalata-mandala* ("forehead circle").

Blocking the ears with their forefingers, the *yogins* can hear the sound *phu* inwardly, and their consciousness space begins to be filled with a phosphorescent bluish light. At the same time a feeling of great bliss suffuses their entire being. This is the first stage of *shambhavi-mudra*, and is known as the "perception of the inner sign" (*antar-lakshya-lakshana*). It is also called *tejo-dhyana* or "fire meditation" in the *Gheranda-Samhita.* The experience is quite transient and needs to be repeated to become established, so that it can be used as a stepping-stone for further efforts on the spiritual path.

The second phase of *shambhavi-mudra* is the "perception of the external sign" (*bahir-lakshya-lakshana*). It is described as the visual experience of an external field of different colors appearing at a distance of between two and six inches from the forehead. It must be understood as a highly dynamic field with waves of blue, red, orange, and similar colors, and with shafts of gold at the fringes. This is experienced with open eyes, and the colorful field is apparently superimposed on the ordinary perceptual image. Thus in the second phase, the internal vision of light is gradually externalized. This technique is said to be perfected when the luminous ether or field is steadily perceived about six inches above the head.

In the third stage of the experiment, the "perception of the intermediate sign" (*madhya-lakshya-lakshana*), everything happens in a greatly intensified manner, and consciousness becomes so absorbed in the experience that one can no longer properly speak of it as a vision or perception. This is *samadhi,* the merging of subject and object. The practitioner *becomes* his or her experiences. The "eternal field" that he or she perceives or, more precisely lives, is both internal and external, and it can assume any of these five forms:

(1) *guna-rabita-akasha:* the ether-space devoid of quality

(2) *parama-akasha:* the supreme ether-space

(3) *maha-akasha:* the great ether-space

(4) *tattva-akasha:* the ether-space of verity

(5) *surya-akasha:* the sun ether-space

These represent distinct experiences associated with specific colors and intensities. Ideally the progression is from the first up to the fifth. This last luminous field is compared to the joint radiance of a hundred thousand suns. On this level the *yogin*'s identification with the "delivering" or *taraka* sign is fully accomplished.

Only one more step remains to be taken, namely the realization of the transmental (*amanaska*) Reality, which is also known as *taraka.* Thus the word *taraka* is used in a double sense. On one hand it refers to the "signs" or visionary experiences induced by *shambhavi-mudra,* and on the other hand it signifies the singular Being itself. This double usage may be misleading for the layman, but to the initiate who has come to understand the nondual basis of existence it is extremely meaningful: The many signs of the unitary Being are not really external to the supreme *taraka* but are merely so many manifestations of it conjured up by the unenlightened mind, which is unable to perceive the highest truth directly.

The transmental *taraka* is synonymous with *nirvikalpa-samadhi*. In this state, the spiritual practitioner *is* the single Being apprehending itself by itself. Here the *yogin*'s inward odyssey finds its fulfillment. Not only is the practitioner's consciousness transmuted into pure Awareness, there seem to be also marked changes in body chemistry. He or she is said to need almost no food, to have conquered sleep, and yet to be strong in body and sound in mind.

The photistic path of *taraka-yoga* utilizes phenomena that were undoubtedly known even in archaic times. We know, for instance, that light phenomena play an important role in Shamanism, which has ancient roots that clearly antedate Yoga. Moreover, the ultimate Reality itself is often called "light" (*jyotis*) in the earliest Vedanta scriptures.

Surprisingly enough, we do not find this usage in the extant works on *taraka-yoga*. Nowhere do they speak of the absolute Reality as being luminous. Instead, it is said to be transmental, that is, transcending the categories of the mind. Thus, it presumably also transcends anything that the mind might experience or conceptualize as "light."

In *taraka-yoga,* experiences of light precede the ultimate realization. Liberation thus implies a leap beyond photisms, indeed beyond any other experiences generated along the yogic path. The transmental (*unmani*) condition reveals the eternal bliss (*ananda*) of the Absolute. However, this bliss is not a content of experience but the very being of the liberated person. As the *Mandala-Brahmana-Upanishad* (II.5.3–4) puts it:

> The *yogins* become that ocean of bliss.

> Compared with that [absolute bliss], Indra and the other [deities] are only moderately blissful. Thus he who has attained [ultimate] bliss is a supreme *yogin*.

16

YANTRA-YOGA: THE PATH OF GEOMETRIC VISUALIZATION

In their endeavor to intensify consciousness and transcend its ordinary limitations, *yogins* have taken advantage of the entire gamut of human expression and potential. Thus, for example, we find that they utilized our capacity for action in *karma-yoga*, our innate devotional ability in *bhakti-yoga*, our ability to produce complex sound patterns in *mantra-yoga*, our faculty of discrimination in *jnana-yoga*, and even our penchant for strong negative emotions like hatred in *samrambha-yoga*.[1] The *yogins* naturally also made use of the most powerful among the senses—the visual sense—in conjunction with our capacity for visualization.

Yogic discipline is essentially a matter of inner focusing. In some schools, this focusing involves actual visualization, or imaging, in which a definite object is held mentally for a prolonged period of time to produce a shift in awareness. Tantrism, for instance, employs geometric designs known as *yantras*, which are considered highly efficient tools of concentration.

According to Tantric philosophy, the many forms in the universe have not only their own distinctive shape perceptible to the physical eye but also their individual "cosmography." That is to say, everything—whether animate or inanimate—carries within itself a faithful "memory tape" of its genesis. Moreover, the story of the cosmos as a whole is also inscribed in it. This is so because even the smallest particles in the cosmos mirror the total structure of the universe. In this sense, every perceptible form can be said to be a *yantra*.

This way of looking at existence is typical of all traditional societies, which regard the world as a sacred event. Traditionally, religion has been a way of acknowledging the fact that there is a link between "Heaven" and Earth. The temples and pyramids of the ancient world were erected to commemorate that connection. It is only in recent centuries that this worldview has been progressively undermined by the ideology of scientism, which seeks to "demythologize" our existence, forgetting that we cannot live by intellect alone.

In their quest for simplicity of understanding and reconnection with the sacred, the metaphysicians of Tantrism arrived at the conclusion that every form in the cosmos can be reduced to a definite number of primary geometrical figures, such as the point, line, triangle, square, and circle. These are thought to have a fixed symbolic value. In combination, they are considered to be expressive of particular qualities as embodied in certain aspects of creation.

In the narrow technical sense, a *yantra* is a complex geometrical pattern specifically employed in Tantrism as an "instrument"—the literal meaning of the word—for internalizing consciousness and transcending the ordinary mind. The *Tantra-Tattva* (folio 519), a late Tantric scripture, states that a *yantra* is so called because it controls (*niyantrana*) the passions and hence also suffering.

A *yantra* is deemed to be a vessel or seat for certain deities representing major creative forces in the universe—such as Lakshmi (who brings good fortune), Vishnu (who pervades all), or the elephant-headed Ganapati or Ganesha (who removes all obstacles).

During a typical Tantric ceremony, these deities are invoked through the recitation of potent sounds (*mantra*), sacred hand gestures, breath control, and a great variety of other ritual techniques. One of the principal practices is to create the respective *yantra* of the deity to be worshipped. This is done by drawing the geometric design on paper or wood or into sand, or by engraving it on metal, or sometimes by modeling it in three dimensions.

But drawing or modeling the *yantra* externally is not enough. Gradually the practitioners of this Yoga must establish the *yantra* within themselves, through intense concentration and visualization. They have to build up a vivid three-dimensional model of the *yantra* within their own minds. Or rather, they must come to realize experientially that their bodies are in truth identical in form with that *yantra*.

This is a very difficult and lengthy process. For us moderns it might even be an impossible task, because we no longer enjoy our ancestors' excellent memory. Traditional societies transmitted their knowledge orally rather than in written form. For instance, the hymns of the Vedas and the verses and prose passages of the Upanishads were originally all memorized, and with astonishing accuracy. However, this wonderful mnemonic gift has been largely lost with the increasingly widespread use of books. But memory is crucial to the kind of visualization called for in Yoga and Tantrism.

The mentally constructed *yantra* must become so vivid that it feels alive. When the practitioners are successful at this inner work, the *yantra* turns into a vibrating force field that completely absorbs their attention. In due course, they can no longer tell whether the *yantra* is within themselves or they are within the *yantra*. Their consciousness is progressively carried into a deep absorption, where they become completely oblivious to their surroundings. Their senses no longer register external stimuli. They live entirely in their inner world. Finally, they become aware of the deity (i.e., the personalized creative force) of the *yantra* itself.

Meditative absorption (*dhyana*) is characterized by a gradual abolition of the subject-object barrier that is fundamental to the ordinary waking consciousness. At the end of the process lies the complete unification of subject and object, the merging of the "knower," the "known," and the act of "knowing." At this point all duality is transcended. This state is called *samadhi*, or "ecstasy."

There are two types of *samadhi*, a "lower" and a "higher." The former has as its base a "form" (*rupa*), or guiding idea, with which the experiencing subject is merging. In the latter type of *samadhi* there is a total absence of contents in consciousness. Consciousness, or rather awareness (*cit*), abides in itself. The empirical consciousness is temporarily abolished, making room for the transcendental "witness" (*sakshin*). This is the condition referred to as Self-realization or liberation.

The meditative experience of the deity of a particular *yantra* belongs to the "lower" mode of *samadhi*. It is considered an invaluable preparation for the ultimate realization of the universal Self.

At the outset of one's practice the *yantra* should, paradoxically, be more complex. Once a certain measure of success in concentration and visualization has been achieved through regular exercise, the *yantra* can be very much simplified. The *yantra* can be internally or externally constructed in two ways. It can be imaged from the innermost point outwards—in accordance with the process of unfoldment of the cosmos. Or it can be imaged from the outermost circumference towards the center—in alignment with the process of meditative absorption. The symbolism of the constituent elements of a *yantra* is comparatively simple. But the inner meaning of a *yantra*, embodied in its deity, can only be fully grasped when it is experienced inwardly.

The principal element of any *yantra*, though not always articulated, is the point or *bindu* ("drop"). It represents that point in space and time where any object comes into manifestation. The *bindu* stands between manifestation and the unmanifest, between actuality and potentiality. It is the creative matrix, the primary structure, from which issues the whole cosmos in its multiformity. This is true both of the physical world and the psychological universe, macrocosm and microcosm.

Manifestation can only occur with movement. Geometrically, this is expressed by a line or a combination of lines. The ascending movement is depicted by an upward pointing triangle, symbolizing the male principle in the universe, or *shiva*. By way of analogy, it is connected with the element of fire and mental activity in general. Its numerical value is 3. The triangle that points downward stands for the female creative principle, or *shakti*, the receptacle of the activity of *shiva*. It is linked with the element of water, and its numerical value is 2.

The dodecagon, one of the more common elements in *yantras*, is

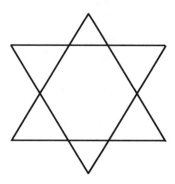

composed of an upward- and a downward-pointing triangle. It symbolizes the state of balance of the manifested world. The existence of the cosmos is made possible by a perfect dynamic equilibrium between opposing forces.

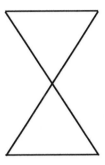

The state of chaos or negation is depicted in the form of two vertically arranged triangles meeting at their tips, thus forming the "drum of Shiva." God Shiva here represents the principle of destruction and thus also of renewal.

The square represents the element of earth (*bhu*); its numerical value is 4. This symbolism is almost universal.

The circle is the symbol of periodicity and rhythm. It can also signify the latent "coiled" energy inherent in matter. It is connected with the fifth element, ether (*akasha*). Its numerical value is 1 or 10 respectively.

The hexagon, as the symbol of the element of air (*vayu*), represents disorderly movement.

The lotuses in various *yantras* signify particular entities or personified energies, which are identifiable by the number of petals. The eight-petaled lotus, for example, is indicative of God Vishnu the preserver.

The Tantric scriptures mention and describe a great number of *yantras*. Most of them are put to spiritual use. But there are some that are employed specifically in order to cure illnesses or to obtain material benefits. The most celebrated *yantra* is undoubtedly the *shri-yantra*, also called the *shri-cakra* ("auspicious wheel"). It is a symbolical archetype of the cosmos and, by way of analogy, of the human body. It is the great symbol of the Goddess (*devi*), or Shakti, both in her transcendental and in her immanent form. *Devi* stands for the female principle in the universe, the power-energy that is responsible for all creation.

According to Tantric philosophy, Goddess and God are really one. Both together constitute or *are* the primordial Unity, the singular Reality beyond all phenomena. Their separation, as experienced on the empirical level, is the reason for all human suffering. Self-realization consists in the discovery that, on the ultimate level of existence, God and Goddess are forever embracing one another, and the Self-realized adept participates in the delight of their eternal union.

The *shri-yantra*, as employed in Tantra liturgy, serves to remind the *yogin* or *yogini* of the ultimate nondifference between subject and object. This *yantra* is composed of nine juxtaposed triangles. These are arranged in such a way that they produce a total of forty-three small triangles. Four of the nine primary triangles point upward, representing the male cosmic energy; five of them point downward, symbolizing the female cosmic power.

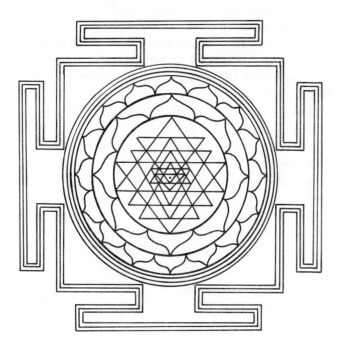

These triangles are surrounded by an eight-petaled lotus symbolizing Vishnu, the all-pervading ascending tendency in the macrocosm and microcosm. The next lotus, with sixteen petals, represents the attainment of the object of desire, particularly the power over the mind and sense-organs. Enclosing this lotus are four concentric lines that are symbolically connected with the two lotuses and the triangles. The triple-line surround is called the "earth-city" (*bhu-pura*); it symbolizes the three spheres of the world, and microcosmically speaking, the human body.

In Southern India, the *shri-yantra* is considered an object of worship. Some of the medieval and later Hindu temples contain shrines in which a smaller altar is to be found. Tradition has it that these altars enshrine engravings of the *shri-yantra*. For reasons of health and, sadly, also for purposes of black magic, the *shri-yantra* is engraved upon a thin gold, silver, or copper foil that is rolled into a cylinder and placed in a metallic case to be worn as a kind of amulet.

A much more detailed pictorial version of the *yantra* is the *mandala*, as used in Tibetan Buddhism (Vajrayana). Instead of a point, imaginary or actually indicated, the *mandala* has as its center the Primeval Buddha from whom proceed in all four directions the "Four Paradises" supervised by various Buddhas, or enlightened beings. Outside the inner "walls" of these paradisiacal fields are the Four Human Buddhas and the Four Guardians.

Yantra-yoga is a form of "inner worship" (*antar-puja*), usually of the Goddess. After the Goddess is invoked through *mantra*, or potent sound, She must be invited into, and properly installed in, the *yantra*, which is Her body. Since the internally visualized *yantra* is none other than the practitioner's own body-mind, the installation of the Goddess means that he or she is now one with Her.

Now begins the still more difficult task of progressively dissolving the *yantra*—proceeding from its outermost to its innermost elements. Since the *yantra* is experienced as one's own body-mind, this dissolution implies the dismantling of one's inner world. When consciousness has been reduced to the absolute zero of the *bindu*, a radical switch occurs. The *yogin* or *yogini* becomes identical with the ultimate Reality, which is superconscious, omnipresent, and eternal. Thus, the *yantra* merely serves as a means of gradually reducing the complexities of the mind until the simplicity of the transcendental Self, or Reality, is recovered. This recovery is enlightenment.

NOTE

1. *Samrambha-yoga*, the "Yoga of hatred," is taught in several of the *Puranas*, which are popular encyclopedic repositories of secular and sacred knowledge. The idea behind this Yoga is that we become what we contemplate. Thus, when hatred becomes an all-absorbing emotion, it focuses the mind. For instance, the *Vishnu-Purana* has the legend of King Shishupala who hated the Divine, in the form of God Vishnu, so intensely that he thought about it all the time and finally became merged with it, achieving spiritual liberation.

17

THE ART OF PURIFICATION (SHODHANA)

A. THE PHILOSOPHY OF PURITY

There are many ways of looking at spiritual life. It has been viewed as a path, a journey, or a ladder to the ultimate Reality. It has also been considered a lifelong discipline, the culture of harmony, the right management of one's energies, or the endeavor to go beyond the "little self" (the ego-identity). Here I propose to examine spiritual life as a comprehensive attempt at purification.

All spiritual traditions regard our ordinary human condition as somehow flawed or corrupt, as falling short of the unsurpassable perfection or wholeness of Reality. As a process of transformation, Yoga endeavors to re-form or even "super-form" the spiritual practitioner. The old Adam has to die before the new super-formed being can emerge—the being who is reintegrated with the Whole.

Not surprisingly, this transmutation of the human personality is also often couched in terms of self-sacrifice. In gnostic terms, the "lower" reality must be surrendered so that the "higher" or divine Reality can become manifest in our lives. For this to be possible, the spiritual practitioner must somehow locate and emulate that higher Reality. He or she must find the "heaven" within, whether by experiential communion or mystical union with the Divine or by an act of faith in which a connection with the Divine is simply assumed until this becomes an actual experience. Spiritual discipline, then, is a matter of constantly "remembering" the Divine, or the transcendental Self.

There can be no such transformation without catharsis, without the shedding of all those aspects of one's being that block our immediate apperception of Reality. Traditions like Yoga and Vedanta can be understood as efforts at progressive "detoxification" of the body-mind, which clears the inner eye so that we can see what is always in front of us—the omnipresent Reality, the Divine. So long as our emotional and cognitive system is toxic or impure, that inner eye remains veiled, and all we see is the world of multiplicity devoid of unity. The modern gnostic teacher Mikhael Aivanhov (1900–1986) remarked about this:

> Not so many years ago, when people's homes were still lit by oil lamps, the glass chimneys had to be cleaned every evening. All combustion produces wastes, and the oil in these lamps deposited a film of soot on the inside of the glass, so that, even if the flame was lit, the lamp gave no light unless the glass was cleaned. The same phenomenon occurs in each one of us, for life is combustion. All our thoughts, feelings and acts, all our manifestations, are the result of a combustion. Now it is obvious that in order to produce the flame, the energy which animates us, something has to burn and that burning necessarily entails waste products which then have to be eliminated. Just as the lamp fails to light up the house if its glass is coated with soot . . . similarly, if a man fails to purify himself he will sink deeper and deeper into the cold and dark and end by losing life itself.[1]

To use another metaphor, Yoga is like an oxygen tank resting at the bottom of a deep and murky pool. Using the tank, we can safely float to the surface. As we ascend, we note that the water gets visibly clearer—the water being a symbol for one's own body-mind. We are immersed in the Divine, but we realize this only when we actively work on purifying our vision.

Patanjali, the founder of Classical Yoga, proffered this important definition of spiritual liberation, the goal of the yogic path: "[The condition of] transcendental 'aloneness' (*kaivalya*) [is attained] when the essence-of-mind (*sattva*) and Self are equal in purity" (*Yoga-Sutra* III.55). The philosophy behind this statement is as follows. The transcendental Self (*purusha*) is inherently pure, perfect. The human mind, which Patanjali here calls *sattva*, is not. By purifying the mind until it becomes as transparent as a mirror, it approximates the eternal purity of the Self, reflecting the Self's natural luminosity and thus assuming the appearance of luminosity itself. In fact, enlightenment is when the mind, or consciousness, reflects the Self's innate lustre without obstruction. This reflected luminosity registers even in the body, and then we speak of "transfiguration," as it occurred in the case of Moses, the prophet Elijah, and not least Jesus of Nazareth.

B. YOGIC TECHNIQUES OF PHYSICAL DETOXIFICATION

The most common Sanskrit term for "purification" is *shodhana*, and for the condition of "purity" it is *shuddhi* or *shauca*. Let us begin with Classical Yoga, which is encoded in Patanjali's *Yoga-Sutra*—a work that probably dates back to the second century A.D. From the *Yoga-Sutra* (II.43), we learn that "through asceticism (*tapas*), owing to the dwindling of impurity, perfection of the body and the sense-organs" is gained.

The practice of *tapas* traditionally includes such exercises as fasting for prolonged periods, standing or sitting stock-still, observing complete silence, or voluntarily exposing oneself to extreme heat or cold, hunger or thirst. These ascetical techniques, which are a part of Patanjali's *kriya-yoga*, have the purpose of steeling the will and cultivating the innate potential of the body-mind. Bodily "perfection," we are told in the *Yoga-Sutra* (III.46), consists in a pleasing physical form, gracefulness, and adamantine robustness.

The ideal of bodily perfection became a prominent theme in the period after Patanjali, especially in the schools of *hatha-yoga,* which has the avowed goal of creating an indestructible "divine body" (*divya-deha*). In the *Yoga-Bija* (51–52), a medieval Sanskrit scripture, we read:

> The body [fashioned through] Yoga is exceedingly strong. Even the deities cannot acquire [such a durable body]. [The *yogin* endowed with such a body] enjoys various supernatural powers and is free from bondage to the body. The body [fashioned through Yoga] is like the sky, nay, even purer than the sky.

To create such a superbody, the *yogin* begins by purifying the physical body. The *Gheranda-Samhita,* a seventeenth-century manual of *hatha-yoga,* lists a large number of such purificatory practices. These are meant to "temper" the body through the "fire of Yoga." Purification is, first of all, accomplished through the "six acts" (*shat-karma*).

These six acts comprise: (1) basic cleansing techniques (*dhauti*), which include such practices as dental care, cleansing of the stomach by different means, and rectal cleansing; (2) water enema and dry enema (*vasti*); (3) nasal cleansing (*neti*) by means of a thin thread; (4) rotation of the vertical abdominal muscles (*nauli*), which is thought to cleanse the stomach and intestines; (5) steady gazing (*trataka*), which is held to purify the eyes; and (6) "skull lustre" (*kapala-bhati*), a form of breathing exercise that is thought to "brighten up" the whole head.

The *Brihad-Yogi-Yajnavalkya*, a medieval work, contains detailed instructions for the ritual of bathing (*snana*), and other scriptures mention still further purificatory practices. All these techniques— some of which are quite dangerous when practiced without expert supervision—are said to cure a variety of diseases. The same claim is made for the different postures (*asana*) and methods of breath control (*pranayama*). The daily ritual bathing, the *Brihad-Yogi-Yajnavalkya* (VII.118 ff.) states, is best done in the early morning in a river connected to the ocean or in the ocean itself. Hot water is said to be useless. Bathing produces mental calm, removes negative emotions, and increases a person's well-being, vitality, and beauty.

This scripture (V.27) further mentions that practitioners who are unable to take their ritual bath because of weakness or time constraints should purify themselves by means of mantra recitation. This is called the "mantric bath" (*mantra-snana*).

Two important yogic means of self-purification are fasting (*upavasa*) and dieting (*ahara*). Fasting has long been known as a highly efficient way of inducing an altered state of consciousness. Abstinence from food changes the chemical composition of the blood, which inevitably has an effect on the mind. But fasting has to be undertaken from the right inner disposition to bear spiritual fruit. Gandhi, who constantly experimented with fasting and strict dieting, observed:

> I am convinced that I greatly benefited by it both physically and morally. But I know that it does not necessarily follow that fasting and similar disciplines would have the same effect for all.

> Fasting can help to curb animal passion, only if it is undertaken with a view to self-restraint . . . if physical fasting is not accompanied by mental fasting, it is bound to end in hypocrisy and disaster.[2]

Already the *Chandogya-Upanishad* (VII.26.2), which belongs to the eighth century B.C., notes the close connection between dietary purity and purity of being. Swami Sivananda of Rishikesh reiterated ancient wisdom when he wrote:

> Mind is formed out of the subtlest portion of food. If the food is impure, the mind also becomes impure. This is the dictum of sages and psychologists.[3]

In other words, food is not merely an aggregate of chemical compounds but contains the quintessence of organic matter, which is the life-force (*prana*). However, while all types of food can be considered a form of *prana,* they are not equally beneficial. Some kinds of food prove more or less toxic to the human system. The Yoga practitioner is therefore very circumspect about his or her nutrition.

The *Bhagavad-Gita* (XVIII.8f.) categorizes food according to the model of the three types of primary constituents (*guna*)— *sattva, rajas,* and *tamas. Sattva* is elevating; *rajas* is aggravating; and *tamas* is sluggish.

> Foods that promote life, lucidity (*sattva*), strength, health, happiness, and satisfaction and that are savory, rich in oil, firm, and heart[-gladdening] are agreeable to the *sattva*-natured [person].

> Foods that are pungent, sour, salty, spicy, sharp, harsh, and burning are coveted by the *rajas*-natured [person]. They cause pain, grief, and disease.

> And [food] that is spoiled, tasteless, putrid, stale, left over, and unclean, is food agreeable to the *tamas*-natured [person].

Not all yogic authorities are in agreement over what constitutes a good diet. However, they all emphasize the importance of dietary restraint (called *mita-ahara*).

From a yogic point of view, illness is the result of an imbalance in the circulation of the life-force. Health must be restored before one can proceed to the higher yogic practices of breath control, sensory withdrawal, concentration, and meditation. Dieting is a key practice in this endeavor of harmonizing the body. Ecstasy (*samadhi*), the final stage of the path of Yoga, is explained as perfect inner balance—a balance that is hard to come by without a healthy body.

The single most important *hatha-yoga* technique of purification is a particular type of breath control that is performed by breathing alternately through the left and the right nostril. This practice is intended to remove all obstructions from the network of subtle channels through which the life-force circulates, thus making proper breath control and deep concentration possible. In the ordinary person, state the scriptures of *hatha-yoga*, the circulation of the life-force is obstructed. The technique of alternate breathing is known as *nadi-shodhana*.

When the subtle conduits (*nadi*) are completely purified, the life-force can circulate freely in the body, and it becomes amenable to voluntary control. Already Patanjali noted in his *Yoga-Sutra* (II.52) that breath control has the effect of removing the "covering" (*avarana*) that prevents one's inner light to manifest clearly.

The objective of *hatha-yoga* is to conduct the life-force along the body's central axis to the crown of the head. This flow of *prana* through the central conduit—called *sushumna-nadi*—is thought to awaken the full psychospiritual potential of the body. This potential is better known as the "serpent power" (*kundalini-shakti*).

✗ When the *kundalini* is awakened from its dormant state in the lowest center (*cakra*) at the base of the spine, it rushes up to the crown center. This ascent is accompanied by a variety of psychic and somatic phenomena. These include visionary states and, when the *kundalini* reaches the top center, ecstatic transcendence into the formless Reality, which is inherently inconceivable and blissful.

As the *kundalini* force is active in the crown center, the rest of the body is gradually depleted of energy. This curious effect is explained as the progressive purification of the five elements (*bhuta*) constituting the physical body—earth, water, fire, air, and ether. The Sanskrit term for this process is *bhuta-shuddhi*.

Purification of the body not only leads to health and inner balance but also affects the way in which a person perceives the world. This is clearly indicated in Patanjali's *Yoga-Sutra* (II.40), which states: "Through purity [the yogin gains] distance from his own limbs [as well as the desire for] noncontamination by others." The decisive phrase *sva-anga-jugupsa* has often been translated as "disgust toward one's own body," but this is not at all in the spirit of Yoga. *Jugupsa* is more appropriately rendered as "distance." The adept is a witness, or an observer, of his or her own bodily structures and processes. In other words, the practitioner's physical being is transparent to him or her.

This attitude is an important antidote against the kind of body narcissism to which *hatha-yoga*, like other systems of body culture, can give rise. Patanjali's aphorism reminds us that the real work is to be accomplished on the spiritual level. Then, as he puts it, the "Seer"—the transcendental Self—will truly shine forth. However, it makes sense to want to enjoy Self-realization in a healthy body, which is the ideal of *hatha-yoga*. This desire need not even be a selfish one, for we could probably serve others more effectively in a healthy body, perhaps even a body endowed with all kinds of extraordinary capabilities (*siddhi*).

C. YOGIC TECHNIQUES OF MENTAL CATHARSIS

Bodily *and* moral purity is fundamental to our physical and mental health. Hence Patanjali's eight-limbed yogic path begins with the ten rules of *yama* and *niyama*, which regulate the social life of Yoga practitioners as well as their relationship to their own body-minds and to the Divine (*ishvara*). Moral and physical purity create the necessary basis for the higher practices of Yoga, which aim at cleansing the mirror of the mind more directly.

Mental purification is accomplished by means of sensory inhibition (*pratyahara*), concentration (*dharana*), meditation (*dhyana*), and ecstatic self-transcendence (*samadhi*). In his *Viveka-Cudamani* (vs. 77), the famous Vedanta master Shankara characterizes objects (*vishaya*) as "poison" (*visha*), because they tarnish consciousness by distracting it from its real task, which is to mirror reality. Our attention is constantly pulled outward by objects, and this externalization of our consciousness prevents us from truly being ourselves. "When the mind pursues the roving senses," states the *Bhagavad-Gita* (II.67), "it carries away wisdom (*prajna*), even as the wind [carries away] a ship on water."

Sense perceptions pollute our inner environment, keeping our mind in a state of turmoil. We are forever hoping for experiences that will make us happy and whole, but our desire for happiness can never be satisfied by external experiences. "Whatever pleasures

spring from contact [with sense objects] are only sources of suffering," declares the *Bhagavad-Gita* (V.22). To find true happiness and
peace, we need to unclutter our mind and remain still. The fatal con-
sequences of focusing on objects rather than the ultimate Subject,
the Self, are described very well in that ancient Yoga scripture
(II.62–63):

> When a man contemplates objects, attachment to them is produced.
> From attachment springs desire [for further contact with the objects]
> and from desire comes anger [when that desire is frustrated].

> From anger arises confusion, from confusion [comes] failure of
> memory; from failure of memory [arises] the loss of wisdom
> (*buddhi*); upon the loss of wisdom, [a person] perishes.

Emotional confusion (*sammoha*) profoundly upsets our cognitive
faculties: We lose our sense of direction, purpose, and identity. The
Sanskrit word for this state is *smriti-bhramsha* or "failure of
memory." When we fail to "recollect" ourselves, wisdom (*buddhi*)
cannot shine forth. But without wisdom, we, as members of the
species *homo sapiens*, are doomed to forfeit not only our status as
human beings but our very life. Spiritual ignorance is binding and
ultimately ruinous. Wisdom can set us free.

In Shankara's *Atma-Bodha* (vs. 16), we read:

> Even though the Self is all-pervading, it does not shine in everything.
> It shines only in the organ-of-wisdom (*buddhi*), like a reflection in a
> clear medium [such as water or a mirror].

The "organ-of-wisdom," which is often called the "higher mind,"
is predominantly composed of *sattva,* the lucidity factor in Nature.
There is a family resemblance between the *sattva* and the Self, and
this curious affinity makes it possible for the Self's radiant presence
to manifest itself to human beings.

The discipline of sensory restraint is crucial to the emergence
of wisdom or gnosis. Without it, concentration and meditation
are impossible. Both these techniques have the purpose of vacating
the inner space so that the "light" of the Self can manifest in full.
Concentration is generally defined in the yogic scriptures as the
"binding" of attention to a single focus. Meditation is the process of
deepening that unfolds on the basis of such concentrated attention.

It reveals more and more "subtle" aspects of one's chosen focus, whether it be a visualized deity or other "prop," a *mantra*, or a locus within one's body.

Ultimately, the knowledge or experiences gained in meditation are considered superior to the knowledge or experiences derived through contact with sense objects. Yet they too must be transcended. Meditation fulfills itself when the meditative consciousness is utterly vacated but lucid. At that point, a significant switch occurs in our awareness. All of a sudden we are fused with the object of contemplation. This is the much-desired state of ecstasy (*samadhi*) in which subject and object are merged and all opposites coincide. In this condition, we bask in the peace and happiness that are an integral part of our authentic nature, the transcendental Self.

However, even in the condition of *samadhi* spontaneous insights (*prajna*) intrude, which are in the final analysis also "impurities." Hence they must likewise be transcended until we have fully recovered our identity as the Self in the extraordinary condition of transconceptual ecstasy (*nirvikalpa-samadhi*). Alas, this ecstatic state is only temporary, and before long our ordinary ego-centric awareness reconstitutes itself. Fortunately, *nirvikalpa-samadhi* (which is also known as *asamprajnata-samadhi* in Classical Yoga) leaves a strong "aftertaste," which can then guide us in our further spiritual adventure.

The remaining challenge is to realize Selfhood in the midst of daily life. This is the ideal of "spontaneous ecstasy" (*sahaja-samadhi*), which is stable and permanent. This sublime condition of enlightenment is the same as "living liberation," about which Shankara says in his *Viveka-Cudamani* (vs. 438):

He who never has the thought of "I" with regard to the body and the senses and the thought of "this" in respect of something different to the "That" [i.e., Reality] is regarded as a [being] who is liberated in life (*jivan-mukta*).

NOTES

1. M. Aivanhov, *Light is a Living Spirit* (Frejus, France: Prosveta, 1987), pp. 91–92.

2. M.K. Gandhi, *An Autobiography: The Story of My Experiments with Truth* (Boston, MA: Beacon Press, 1957), p. 332.

3. Swami Sivananda, *Practice of Yoga* (Sivanandanagar, India: Divine Life Society, 1970), p. 214.

18

WHAT IS MEDITATION?

When we examine the quite extensive literature on meditation, we find that meditation has been explained in many different ways. Here are some of the explanations I encountered while writing this essay:

> Meditation is a method by which a person concentrates more and more upon less and less. The aim is to empty the mind while, paradoxically, remaining alert. [1]

> The concept "meditation" refers to a set of techniques which are the production of another type of psychology, one that aims at personal rather than intellectual knowledge. As such, the exercises are designed to produce an alteration in consciousness—a shift away from the active, outward-oriented, linear mode and toward the receptive and quiescent mode, and usually a shift from an external focus of attention to an internal one. [2]

> Meditation is a procedure that allows one to investigate the process of one's own consciousness and experiencing, and to discover the more basic, underlying qualities of one's existence as an intimate reality. [3]

> Meditation . . . is a deliberate switching-off of these external stimuli that prepare the nervous system for fight or flight, and a courting of the heretofore unconscious stimuli which have hitherto been reduced to a minimum by the process of individual selective awareness. [4]

> Basically, meditation can be described as any discipline that aims at enhancing awareness through the conscious directing of attention. [5]

It is evident from the above explanations that meditation is a complex phenomenon that can be viewed from many different angles. Each explanation both reveals and obscures. In the final analysis, it proves to be an elusive, even mysterious process.

While we can meaningfully talk about meditation, just as we can talk about love or life itself, we have to meditate, live, and love in order to truly understand what is meant by these things. In this essay I will talk about meditation, basing myself principally on the sacred literature of Hinduism and, secondarily, on my own experience as a meditator. Specifically, I will make use of the *Rig-Veda*, some of the *Upanishads*, the *Bhagavad-Gita*, the *Yoga-Sutra*, and some of the scriptures on *hatha-yoga*.

Beginning with the meditation practices described in the ancient *Vedas* well over three thousand years ago: As the British Vedicist Jeanine Miller has shown, the bards (*rishi*) who composed the Vedic hymns were not merely inspired poets but *seers*; they claimed to have *seen* the hymns.[6] Then they *sang* what had been revealed to them in their visions. Thus, the Vedic hymns are, by and large, songs of praise used during various ritual occasions.

The visions of these seer-bards are called *dhi*. This word is derived from the same root that also yielded the word *dhyana*, which is the most common designation for "meditation" in the Sanskrit language.

The *rishis* gave their meditative activity the technical designation *brahman*, a word they derived from the verbal root *brih*, meaning "to grow, expand." *Brahman*, in the ancient Vedic sense, is the magical act of "drawing forth" sacred power from the psyche. It is, as Miller explained, a recapitulation of the cosmogonic process itself. The seer's *brahman* duplicates, psychologically, the genesis of the universe itself, which emerged from the transcendental Reality, which is neither being nor nonbeing.

In this meditative state, illumined vision (*dhi*) occurs. Through *brahman*, which is always "god-given" (*devattam*), the "sun" is made manifest. That is to say, meditation manifests splendorous light of the transcendental Reality, the luminous superconsciousness, which was later called *cit*. The Vedic seers knew that the effulgence of stars and the radiance to be discovered in the heart are aspects of the same principle.

Miller distinguished three types of *brahman* meditation:

1. *mantric meditation*, or the absorption of attention in and through sound (*mantra*);

2. *visual meditation,* or the generation of illumined thought (*dhi*) during which a particular deity is invoked;

3. *absorption in mind and heart,* or the deepening of meditation by pondering the illumined insight (*dhi* or *manisha*) further.

The Vedic seers themselves also knew of a "fourth *brahman,*" which Miller identified as the ecstatic state beyond meditation. It is in this fourth *brahman* that the seers experienced great joy and freedom from fear, as well as "immortality" (*amrita*).

The Vedic notion of meditation is associated with a number of other key concepts, notably *hrid* ("heart"), *tapas* ("flame-power"), *kratu* ("creative will"), and *rita* ("truth" or "cosmic order"). The heart stands for inwardness, our inner life, as concentrated in the faculty of higher feeling, which has anciently been connected with the physical heart. The heart is the "cave" in which the hidden treasure may be found—an almost universal idea in the religious traditions of the world.

Tapas, again, is generally rendered as "asceticism," but has far deeper connotations. It is first and foremost the inner glow and power achieved through utmost self-discipline, and it corresponds to the self-confinement exercised by the primordial Being in producing the multifarious universe. The ascetic's *tapas* is, in other words, an exact symbolic duplication of the Creator's original act of self-sacrifice, which alone brought forth the cosmos.

Self-discipline is not so much a matter of negation as the creative channeling of primal energies. This idea is captured in the word *kratu,* often translated as "will." *Kratu* is the psychological power behind the incredible work of *tapas.* It is the will to bring what is originally invisible into the visible realm, so that it can be understood. The visions of the Vedic *rishis* are the product of their inner determination to create.

Such creation always follows universal laws, and the resultant visions are expressions of the cosmic order (*rita*). Conforming to the invisible order of the universe, they render the divine truth tangible. The *rishis* are, therefore, conveyors of the truth, the primordial harmony, underlying all appearances. We can appreciate the immense richness of the Vedic seers' spiritual understanding of life.

The considerable wealth of their religious and mystical ideas was increased in subsequent times. From about the ninth century B.C. onward, the Hindu sages composed the *Upanishads*. These are esoteric explanations and expositions of the Vedic lore, but in many ways they represent a new orientation. In keeping with this change, meditation was henceforth called *dhyana*. We also find in the *Upanishads* the earliest references to the tradition of Yoga, which gradually evolved into the "six-limbed" (*shad-anga*) and then the "eight-limbed" (*ashta-anga*) path.

Moreover, the Vedic key word *brahman* now acquired a new meaning. From then on it referred no longer to the state of meditation but to the Divine or ultimate Reality itself, signifying the great powerful expanse of the sacred. As the core of the psyche or mind, that same Reality came to be known as the "Self" (*atman*).

In the *Chandogya-Upanishad* (VII.6.1), one of oldest of these scriptures, we find a most interesting passage, which provides an important clue about meditation. It reads:

> Meditation (*dhyana*), assuredly, is more than thought. The Earth meditates, as it were (*iva*). The atmosphere meditates, as it were. Heaven meditates, as it were. The waters meditate, as it were. Mountains meditate, as it were. Gods and men meditate, as it were. Hence those among men here who attain greatness—they are, as it were, a part of the estate of meditation. Now, those who are small are quarrelers, maligners, slanderers. But those who are superior—they are, as it were, a part of the estate of meditation. [Therefore,] value meditation.

What does all this mean? First of all, we are told that meditation is more than "thought." The Sanskrit text uses the word *citta* here, which, we are told in the preceding passage, is more than "intention" (*samkalpa*), which, in turn, is more than "intellection" (*manas*). *Citta* probably signifies here ordinary consciousness. Thus, meditation is "more than" the average consciousness. In fact, it is a higher form of awareness.

But why does the anonymous author state that "the Earth meditates, as it were"? Or that "mountains meditate, as it were"? The phrase "as it were" (*iva*) makes it clear that he did not want us to think that the mountains were engaged in a deliberate exercise.

Nevertheless, he insisted, they were engaged in something resembling meditation.

If you have ever taken a leisurely hike in the countryside with no worries on your mind, simply experiencing the hills, trees, and brooks, you will no doubt have been struck by their stillness, their utmost simplicity. They simply abide without any concerns or problems. This is exactly the condition of meditation. Meditation is simply being present as the hills, trees, and brooks are present.

Meditation is abiding. The old word "abide" comes from the Anglo-Saxon *bidan* meaning "to wait." Meditation is indeed a kind of waiting, though not the semiconscious, nervous waiting that typically happens when we stand at a bus stop or sit in the reception area of a dentist's office. Meditative waiting is resting in the present, without the usual flight into thought. It is "just sitting," as the Zen Buddhists put it. Meditation is thus a form of centering, which involves our disengagement from the machine of the mind and our resting in the heart.

The Upanishadic sages preserved many of the Vedic spiritual motifs. Thus they placed the Self in the heart. One of the Sanskrit words for "heart" is *hridaya*. In the *Chandogya-Upanishad* (VIII. 3.3), the word is fancifully explained as "that which is in the heart" (*hridy ayam*), meaning the Self.

By practicing the "friction" of meditation, one may see the "resplendent deity" (*deva*) who is hidden within the heart, declares the *Shvetashvatara-Upanishad* (I.14). This practice is done by using the body as the lower friction-stick and the syllable *om* as the upper friction-stick. Through the combined action of the two "sticks" the spiritual fire is kindled. This notion takes us back to the Vedic *tapas*, which includes an element of tension or friction as well. Through "glow" of *tapas*, the ascetic supercharges his or her body with transformative energy, which, in the end, yields the desired meditative vision of the Divine.

Some time during the fifth or fourth century B.C. the *Bhagavad-Gita* was composed. This wonderful scripture is deemed an honorary *Upanishad*. The word *dhyana* occurs many times in this work, as does the term *yoga*. In fact, the sixth chapter bears the title *Dhyana-Yoga*, and verses 10 to 15 offer a summary of the meditative approach taught by the God-man Krishna, the spiritual hero of the *Gita.*

In verse XII.12, again, *dhyana* is said to be better than wisdom (*jnana*), but then renunciation is said to be better than meditation, because it leads straightaway to peace. However, this verse can also be read differently and more convincingly as stating that renunciation springs from meditation, and from renunciation comes peace.

In the *Gita,* the God-man Krishna asks his disciple Arjuna to yoke his "wisdom-faculty" (*buddhi*) by fastening it on him. In this way the entire body-mind becomes focused as well. Krishna speaks of those who have renounced all actions in him and who are intent on him alone, worshipping him by contemplating (*dhyai*) him through the practice of Yoga. This is an early statement of the practice of *guru-yoga,* where the adept-teacher serves as a focal point for the disciple's meditative and devotional life. The underlying idea is that the Self-realized master is a doorway to the Divine.

In the *Maitrayaniya-Upanishad* (VI.18), which dates back to the second or third century B.C., we find the first formulation of the yogic path as a process of clearly demarcated stages, called "limbs" (*anga*). This scripture enumerates them as follows: breath control (*pranayama*), sensory inhibition (*pratyahara*), meditation (*dhyana*), concentration (*dharana*), appraisal (*tarka*), and ecstasy (*samadhi*)—in this order. Thus meditation appears as the third "limb." It is unclear why concentration succeeds rather than precedes it, though perhaps this is a hint at the fact that concentration and meditation are closely linked inner processes.

The practice of *tarka,* here translated as "appraisal," is not explained in the *Maitraniya-Upanishad.* However, it likely refers to the exercise of careful examination of the quality and effects of one's meditation. Without self-criticism, the moods and visions engendered by meditation can become obstacles to the spiritual process. The Yoga practitioners must apply discrimination to their life as a whole, but especially to the manifestations of their own psyches. As the contemporary philosopher-sage Paul Brunton put it:

> Meditation must be accompanied by constant effort in the direction of honest self-examination. All thoughts and feelings which act as a barrier between the individual and his Ultimate Goal must be overcome.

This requires acute self-observation and inner purification . . . He must be on his guard against the falsifications, the rationalizations, and the deceptions unconsciously practised by his ego when the self-analysis exercises become uncomfortable, humiliating, or painful. Nor should he allow himself to fall into the pit of self-pity.[7]

Formulations like those of the *Maitrayaniya-Upanishad* prepared the way for the classical eightfold path of Patanjali, who probably lived in the second century A.D. In Patanjali's school, meditation figures as the seventh "limb." It is immediately preceded by the practice of concentration and succeeded by ecstasy. The fact that there are these stages reminds us that meditation is not an end in itself. It is simply a means to Self-realization through the mediating practice of ecstatic self-transcendence.

It is very important to realize that meditation is an integral part of the spiritual path. This means it cannot be practiced successfully apart from the other "limbs." Moreover, *dhyana* is not a self-contained state, but its thrust is toward its own transcendence, that is, toward ecstasy, or *samadhi*. *Dhyana* makes no sense outside the context of enlightenment, or spiritual liberation.

How did Patanjali explain *dhyana*? In aphorism III.2, he tells us that "meditation is the one-directional-flow of the presented-idea with regard to the [object of meditation]." We cannot understand this rather technical aphorism in isolation. It refers back to concentration. In fact, we cannot understand the meditative process according to Patanjali without going still further back, namely to the practice of posture (*asana*). Meditation really starts there. For, posture involves a high degree of relaxation and, as Patanjali puts it in aphorism II.47, one's "coinciding with the infinite [space of consciousness]."

This practice induces a measure of insensitivity to external stimuli, thus naturally leading over into the practice of sensory withdrawal (*pratyahara*) followed by concentration and meditation.

In aphorism II.11, which is often glossed over by readers of the *Yoga-Sutra,* Patanjali tells us another very important fact about meditation. He states that "the fluctuations of these [causes-of-suffering] are to be overcome by meditation." In other words, meditation rather than ecstasy is the means of transcending the mind's perpetual fluctuations (*vritti*).

The fluctuations, again, are merely one of the aspects of the "causes-of-suffering" (*klesha*), namely spiritual ignorance, the sense of individuality, the thirst for life, passionate attachment to beings and things, and the emotion of aversion. Another, subtler, aspect of the "causes-of-suffering" comprises the special mental acts associated with the lower stages of ecstasy, which are distinct from ordinary thoughts. At any rate, the ecstatic state cannot even occur until the *vrittis* have been brought under control in meditation!

The specific task of the different forms of "conscious ecstasy" (*samprajnata-samadhi*), composing the lower level of ecstasy, is to get the "presented-ideas" (*pratyaya*) under control. These are spontaneous thought forms, higher types of insight (*prajna*), arising in the ecstatic state. They need to be transcended so that the condition of supraconscious ecstasy (*asamprajnata-samadhi*) can come about.

We may note here that, for Patanjali, any locus (*desha*) is as good as any other for focusing the mind and achieving the meditative state. His broad-minded attitude permitted the elaboration of meditation techniques in subsequent times. One of these later developments represents the typical meditation practice in *hatha-yoga*, which is a complex *visualization* technique. Just how complex this meditation can be is best illustrated by the following passage from the *Gheranda-Samhita* (VI.2–8):

> [Let the *yogin*] visualize that there is a great sea of nectar in his own heart; that in the middle of that [sea] there is an island of precious stones, the sand of which [consists of] pulverized gems; that on all sides of it are *nipa* trees laden with sweet blossoms; that next to these trees, like a rampart, there is a row of flowering trees such as *malati, mallika, jati, kesara, campaka, parijata,* and *padma,* and that the fragrance of their blossoms is spreading all round in every direction. In the middle of this garden, let the *yogin* visualize that there is a beautiful *kalpa* tree with four branches, representing the four *Vedas,* and that it is laden with blossoms and fruits. Beetles are humming there and cuckoos are singing. Beneath that [tree] let him visualize a great platform of precious gems. Let the *yogin* [further] visualize that in its center there is a beautiful throne inlaid with jewels. On that [throne] let the *yogin* visualize his particular deity (*devata*), as taught by the teacher [who will instruct him about] the appropriate form, adornment, and vehicle of that deity. Know the constant meditation of such a form to be "coarse meditation" (*sthula-dhyana*).

Meditation, often of the visualizing variety, has also been a part of the Western religious and esoteric traditions. Often it took the form of prayer and visualization combined, as in the case of the "heart prayer" of the Eastern Church. Christian monastics also used *mantras* like "Hail Mary" in their meditative practice. But these efforts never produced a system of meditation that was as intricate as those we encounter in the Hindu and Buddhist literature. Nevertheless, practitioners of Eastern meditation techniques can certainly benefit from studying Christian approaches. Conversely, spiritual seekers adopting Christian forms of prayer and meditation are clearly able to enrich their practice by a close study of Eastern methods.

Today the West is pioneering the scientific exploration of meditation. This interest was chiefly initiated by practitioners of Transcendental Meditation (TM), the meditation system developed by Maharishi Mahesh Yogi. It seems fitting, therefore, to comment briefly on this particular approach. Despite all the secrecy surrounding it, TM is really a form of *mantra-yoga,* supposedly the simplest type of Yoga. Initiates are given, usually for a hefty fee, their own specific *mantra* taken from a limited pool of such "words of power" as *om, ram,* or *ham.* They are then asked to focus their attention on and through that sacred sound during each meditative session.

Many claims have been made about TM, ranging from simple physiological effects to extraordinary parapsychological phenomena. One of the more interesting, if controversial, claims concerns the "field effect" of meditation. It is said that TM is an effective means of improving the psychic environment of the world, capable of preventing war and other similar disasters. As any meditator can confirm, the meditative state not only has a benign effect on his or her own inner environment but *can* also extend to other beings who are directly exposed to the meditator's peaceful presence. How far-reaching this effect is, however, and how it functions, remain to be fully investigated.

Psychologists have succeeded in giving us a fairly good picture of what happens physiologically and psychologically in meditation. They have shown that meditation is an unusual but largely beneficial condition. They have also given us all kinds of operational facts about it, such as the correlation that exists between certain levels of meditative experiencing and brain waves. In fact, this discovery has led to a whole new technology, known as "biofeedback," which has the purpose of facilitating the induction of brain waves characteristic of relaxation and meditation.

The usefulness of this technology still needs to be demonstrated. Above all, we must realize that it can never be a substitute for spiritual maturation. While we may trick our nervous system into functioning in certain ways by wiring ourselves to sophisticated gadgetry, there is no real shortcut on the path to enlightenment.

In the final analysis, for meditation to promote our quest for personal wholeness it must be integrated with a sound spiritual orientation and overall discipline. Genuine meditation practice always unfolds in the context of our encounter with the sacred dimension, and this necessarily involves the transcendence of the ego or, in old-fashioned terms, self-surrender.

NOTES

1. J.H. Clark, *A Map of Mental States* (London: Routledge & Kegan Paul, 1983), p. 29.

2. R.E. Ornstein, *The Psychology of Consciousness* (San Francisco: W.H. Freeman, 1972), p. 107.

3. J. Welwood, ed., *The Meeting of the Ways: Explorations in East/West Psychology* (New York: Schocken Books, 1979), p. 117.

4. C.M. Cade and N. Coxhead, *The Awakened Mind: Biofeedback and the Development of Higher States of Awareness* (Longmead, England: Element Books, 1987), p. 95.

5. D. Goleman, "Meditation: Doorway to the Transpersonal," in R.N. Walsh and F. Vaughan, eds., *Beyond Ego: Transpersonal Dimensions in Psychology* (Los Angeles: J.P. Tarcher, 1980), p. 136.

6. See J. Miller, *The Vedas: Harmony, Meditation and Fulfilment* (London: Rider, 1974).

7. P. Brunton, *The Notebooks of Paul Brunton*, vol. 4, part 1: *Meditation* (Burdett, NY: Larson Publications, 1986), pp. 172–173.

19

SILENCE IS GOLDEN: THE PRACTICE OF MAUNA

Most of us know the age-old saying, "Speech is silvern, silence is golden." But what does it mean? We seldom reflect on our ancient wisdom anymore, and so we fail to notice many useful things that people were once taught by their elders.

On one level, the maxim quoted above simply means that silence is better than speech. But, as I will show, there is another, deeper, meaning to it. Let's begin with the obvious, however. Why should silence be better than speech? When we speak, after all, we communicate with others, which is to say, we are in relationship. Silence, on the other hand, causes awkwardness and can be misunderstood. At least, this is how one might view the situation.

But how often do we communicate falsehoods in our speech? Or how frequently do we fail to communicate adequately? That is, how often do we misunderstand each other as a result of the spoken word? The answer is: most of the time. You can easily test this fact by playing a party game, which could be called "rumor": Whisper a message in someone's ear. That person has to pass the message on to the next person, and so on. By the time the message reaches you again, you will be surprised to find how little is left of your original message. Speech frequently distorts information, because the speaker seldom pays attention to what he or she is saying, and the listener generally is listening with only one ear.

Sacred speech stands in striking contrast to casual speech. In sacred speech, both speaker and listener are attentive to what is being communicated. Hence in the spiritual traditions of humanity, which originally were oral traditions, the sacred teachings have been remarkably well preserved from generation to generation. Memorization was a sacred art and obligation. The invention of books has undermined this art.

We may recall here the primary meaning of the Greek word *mythos*, which stands for the sacred utterance or story told by the tribal elder who had been initiated into the secrets of life. This word stems from the verb *mytheomai*, meaning "to talk, to speak." But, significantly, its root *mu* has yielded another word, *myein*, which means "to close." Thus, myth implies both the closing, or guarding, of the mouth in order to receive the inner, visionary revelation, and the opening of the mouth in order to communicate that revelation.

Silence is, of course, also a kind of communication. Therefore it can be either understood correctly or misinterpreted. People are silent for a large number of reasons: to withhold information, to feel superior, to repress their feelings, to stand off from a difficult situation, to underscore what they have just said, to communicate feelings with their eyes or other parts of their bodies, to feel more intensely, to express disapproval, and so on.

But there is another kind of silence, which, in India, is known as *mauna*. This Sanskrit word is generally translated as "silence," but it conveys much more to native speakers of Sanskrit. It stems from the same verbal root as the word *manas*, meaning "mind." The root is *man*, meaning "to ponder" but also "to meditate." *Mauna* is not simply "thinking." On the contrary, it is the absence of thought, while being intensely present in the inner environment. *Mauna* is sacred silence. It is meditation.

The practitioner of *mauna* is called a *muni*. Now, a muni is never described as an individual who is merely silent. Rather, he is known as an ecstatic. Thus we may ask: What have sacred silence and ecstasy in common? In sacred silence, we transcend our human condition. We stand (*stasis*) outside (*ex*) our ordinary egoic personality. This self-transcendence fulfills itself in the state of ecstasy, in which our psychic conditioning is temporarily suspended in utter bliss.

The spiritual discipline of silence—and it is a discipline or a voluntary self-chastening—is thus not merely the absence of speech or utterance. What appears from the outside to be a negative condition is inwardly experienced as an immense richness, or fullness. For the discipline of silence is practiced not only in regard to the organ of speech, but also in regard to the mind itself. It includes the silencing of the mental chatter that characterizes the ordinary person. This deep inner silence is experienced as peace and, ultimately, as an abundance of bliss. As the British essayist Thomas Carlyle, in his work *Sartor Resartus* (1834), put it: "Silence is the element in which great things fashion themselves together."

Sacred silence, then, is an activity that is really a counteractivity, for it engenders stillness. It *is* stillness. And that stillness opens up the dimension of spiritual existence—that luminous world that awaits our discovery as soon as we redirect our attention from external things to our own radiant depths. In the *Isha-Upanishad* (vs. 17), an esoteric Hindu text composed in the centuries before Christ, the anonymous author prays:

> The face of Truth is covered with a golden lid. Remove it, O Fosterer,
> for him who adheres to the Truth.

Sacred silence leads to and beyond the lustrous "golden orb" in the nucleus of our own being. Through silence, we traverse the bright inner dimensions until we penetrate to the blinding Light of the ultimate Reality itself, and become one with It. *So'ham*, "I am He," declare the Upanishadic sages in their rapture.

In many spiritual traditions, this transcendental Reality is symbolized by the sun. The reason for this is not far to seek: Like the sun, the transcendental Reality is experienced by the mystics of all ages as life-giving and radiant. It *is* Life itself. As one Upanishadic sage put it long ago, it is by the power of that Reality that the sun and all the myriad other stars do their work.

Silence is not merely a discipline; rather, it is primarily a state of being. It is in, through, and as silence that we discover our authentic identity, the Self (*atman, purusha*). Thus silence partakes of the golden nature of the ultimate Reality. By comparison, speech is like the silver-bodied moon, which has no light of its own but is illuminated by the radiance of the sun.

Through silence we can attune ourselves to the supreme stillness of the single Being, which is utter silence that is never disrupted by sound. Jean Klein, a contemporary exponent of Advaita Vedanta, comments:

> The Self is silent awareness and cannot be defined in terms of a silence as opposed to noise. How should we react towards silence or its opposite? If you want to rid yourself of agitation so as to attain a state of silence, you reject, you fight, you defend yourself. But if on

the contrary you were to accept it, the agitation—which is part of this silence—will disappear within it. Then you will reach the silence of the Self, beyond silence and agitation.[1]

Once that great, sustaining Reality has been discovered, all our actions, thoughts, and utterances become spontaneous signals of that infinite silence, which is sheer bliss. Thus, the words of the enlightened adepts have transformative power, because they address that part in us which instinctively knows of that unsurpassed silence.

Just as in ordinary life, speech and silence are intimately interwoven, so also in spiritual life do they complement one another. This has been recognized particularly in Taoism. In the language of the *I Ching*, speech is the *yang* or masculine pole of silence, and silence is the *yin* or feminine pole of speech. Together they are responsible for the creativity of human interaction. In spiritual life we cultivate sacred silence to regenerate our inner being so that we can return to our daily activities and to speech from a new perspective.

In his monumental *Study of History*, the great British historian Arnold Toynbee has written about the creative withdrawal of the spiritual heroes of the past—the founders and inspirers of religions. They sought out the wilderness in order to find the fountain of truth within their own being. Then they returned, strengthened and ready to uplift humanity by sharing with others their extraordinary discovery.

We need not have the spiritual stature of a Moses, Jesus, Mahavira, or Gautama the Buddha to practice sacred silence, and benefit from it. "Silence," said Ovid, "is strength."

NOTE

1. J. Klein, *Neither This Nor That I Am* (London: Watkins, 1981), p. 90.

20

SEX, ASCETICISM, AND MYTHOLOGY

Friedrich Nietzsche, the nineteenth-century German philosopher who defiantly declared the death of God, once remarked that the human being is a rope stretched between animal and deity. He could as easily have likened us to the tension between sex hormones and higher cerebral impulses. Nietzsche's metaphor, like most metaphors, is only partly to the point. For, in a very real sense, we also *are* our genitals just as we *are* our brain and all the other aspects of our bodily being. And, needless to say, we are a great deal more, as serious practitioners of different spiritual disciplines throughout the ages have discovered for themselves.

Nevertheless, mastering the dynamic between biological needs—specifically, genital urges—and higher evolutionary or transpersonal aspirations is a crucial part of all moral, religious, and spiritual traditions of the world. Typically we experience these two sets of wants or needs as being at war with each other: Don't let the cerebrum know what the genitals are doing. Suppress your desires. Curb your sexual curiosity. Feel ashamed about having genitals.

This body- and sex-negative orientation is epitomized in the religious doctrine according to which the "flesh" is the enemy of the "spirit." For love to be "pure," it must be devoid of sexual connotations. At best, sex is regarded as a necessary evil. As the British mathematician-philosopher Bertrand Russell observed, this view has caused millions of people great misery. For they had to suppress their sexual instincts in the hope of a better life in the hereafter, where, as sexless (possibly even disembodied) angelic beings, they could participate in the joys of heaven beyond all genitality and sexual complications.

This dualistic idea, which splits the human being into genital or sensual and spiritual or ascetical compartments, is at home in Christianity as much as it is in Islam, Hinduism, and Buddhism. For instance, the ancient *Rig-Veda*, the Old Testament of Hinduism, records a domestic quarrel between the sage Agastya and his wife Lopamudra. The cause of their quarrel was—of course—sex. Agastya, who was a renowned ascetic and a paragon of the virtue of chastity, was, frankly, neglecting his wife. In other words, he preferred meditating in solitude over making love to her. Understandably, she was beginning to feel frustrated. So, she started to complain and make demands.

At first, the sage valiantly defended his position. No doubt, his wife would have expected no less of him. Lopamudra, who knew her husband well, was not inexperienced in the art of seduction. Bit by bit, Agastya succumbed to her womanly wiles. No sooner had he broken his vow of sexual abstinence than he felt great compunction. To "purify" himself again, he made all kinds of sacrificial offerings to the gods. Probably a very happy Lopamudra was aiding him in his rituals.

We may speculate that the intimate conversation between the couple found its way into the most venerated part of the sacred literature of the Hindus because it described a common situation in ancient times: a householder-ascetic struggling with his own and his wife's sexuality in the midst of a demanding spiritual life. This struggle, which has brought many would-be ascetics to their knees, has been fought by men and women ever since religions began to propagandize the idea that in order to fulfill spiritual life one must curb the passions of the flesh. Whole traditions arose that were based on this mistaken idea—namely, that communion with the Divine, or God-realization, depends on repressing, confining, or somehow "sublimating" the sexual urge.

Certainly, utter renunciation of sex was the grand ideal to which countless ascetics in ancient India aspired. Many of them came to be remembered in the popular and sacred literature. A good many, however, are remembered for failing to uphold this supreme ideal. Thus, the *Mahabharata,* one of India's two national epics, is filled with tales of fallen ascetics. A favorite story-telling motif is that of a particularly zealous penitent being sorely tempted by an unearthly damsel, sent by one of the gods to test the ascetic's determination and patience.

In the *Ramayana*, the second and older national epic, we hear of the illustrious sage Vishvamitra whose passion was inflamed when he saw beautiful Menaka bathe naked in a stream near his hermitage. His love affair with her lasted for a full ten years, at which point he "came to his senses" and resumed, with doubly fierce resolution, his ascetic mode of life.

Sharadvant, a mighty *yogin* and skilled archer, was tested in a similar fashion. When he spotted a scantily clad maiden, he temporarily lost control over his mind, stood agape, and involuntarily dropped his bow and arrows, as well as his semen. The famous sages Vyasa, Kashyapa, Bharadvaja, Mankanaka, and Dadhica experienced similar mishaps.

For the male ascetic, lust is the ally of death. The reason for this is that the loss of semen signals to him the loss of power, energy, and hard-earned merit. The ascetic needs good merit to cheat the iron law of karma, and he requires the body's energy to accomplish the magnificent work of self-transformation that is the goal of all austerities. The ascetic is a hoarder of psychosomatic energy. He guards all bodily openings, especially the genitals. Semen is, for him, not merely semen but a substance of power that must be accumulated, not squandered. The typical ascetic is always worrying about the involuntary loss of semen, or becoming sexually aroused to the point where he loses control over his thoughts.

That chastity is not to be confused with self-emasculation is a point made in many of the stories: Whenever a *yogin* has been distracted from his single-minded discipline, he proves to be a most virile and vigorous lover. In India, it is well known that *yogins* acquire great sexual attractiveness, and that this is one of the dangers lurking on the spiritual path. This is why not a few Western ladies swoon over their favorite swami, often without understanding that the secret of his sexual attractiveness lies in his prolonged sexual abstinence. Little wonder that *yogins* and *yoginis* have from time immemorial been warned to steer clear of the other sex. But this traditional warning merely plays into the body-negative inclinations of many ascetics, and it encourages "spiritual narcissism" rather than the enlightened attitude of love and compassion.

That male ascetics are not eunuchs is best exemplified in the person of Shiva, the destroyer aspect of the Hindu trinity of gods. He is both ascetic and sex fiend *par excellence*. Shiva's dual nature is brought out beautifully in the *Puranas*, India's traditional encyclopedia-like compilations in Sanskrit, which contain numerous myths, legends, and philosophical as well as theological accounts. The following is a story from the *Skanda-Purana*, which portrays the divine Shiva sporting a range of very human character traits.

> Shiva played dice with his celestial spouse, Parvati, who beat him by cheating. Angry at having lost, Shiva started a noisy quarrel. To cool his temper, which threatened to upset whole worlds, he took to the forest. In the manner of a true ascetic, he stripped off all his clothes and enjoyed the solitude
>
> Parvati, however, felt twinges of guilt about her cheating and also was filled with longing for her husband. Taking a friend's good advice, she decided to ask for his forgiveness. She assumed the form of a most beautiful maiden, magically transported herself into the forest, and appeared before Shiva.
>
> The great lord of *yogins* was stirred from his meditation. When he saw the voluptuous damsel, he was instantly filled with desire. He reached out for her, but she promptly vanished into thin air. Tormented by his lust for that mysterious beauty, Shiva took to wandering. Then one day he encountered her again. This time he was careful to approach her with less impetuousness. The maiden told him that she was in search of a husband who is all-knowing and in control of his emotions. Without batting an eyelid, Shiva volunteered himself immediately. However, the beauty told him that he could not possibly be qualified to be her husband, since he had abandoned his wife, Parvati, whose love he had won by his excessive austerities. Shiva denied this charge.
>
> Then, changing her tactics, the maiden hailed him as the lord of ascetics and the master of the god of passion. Shiva's response to this was to attempt to take the girl by force. She

demanded to be released at once, and firmly instructed him to ask her father for permission first. Shiva consented. The maiden's father failed to understand how the lord of the universe could possibly be so captivated by, and deluded about, any woman, however lovely. This provoked the sage Narada to poke fun at Shiva, observing that contact with women always makes men ridiculous.

Narada's words made their point. Shiva suddenly realized his wife's charade. He roared with laughter. But then he set out to perform fierce austerities that would make all beings tremble in fear. Parvati then assumed her real form and, prostrating herself before the mighty God, asked him for forgiveness. Shiva was appeased by this gesture and returned to his celestial abode with her—no doubt to resume his eternal play as well as intermittent domestic quarrels with Parvati.

This story, like so many others, depicts Shiva as a figure full of contradictions. He is the supreme deity, and yet he commits the all-too-human folly of lusting after a girl whose beauty is by all appearances as ephemeral as any mortal being's. He is capable of the most intense ascetic fervor and at the same time falls prey to the very desire that he once conquered in the form of Kama, the God of Desire. He takes himself very seriously, and then again he can break into cosmic laughter over his seeming lapse of divine stature. He assumes the role of a fool who can be tricked at dice, but he is the omniscient, all-powerful Lord of Creation who, by a single intention, can plunge the universe into nothingness.

Judged by mortal standards, Shiva is an impossibility. But, then, Shiva is not subject to mortality or human-made standards. He *is* all possibilities of life at once. He is life. As such, Shiva is an instructive symbol for the spiritual practitioner who senses that one can embrace a discipline of self-transcendence without having to turn one's back on life.

Shiva's eroticism is a slap in the face for all those ascetics who associate their personal salvation with sexual sublimation or, worse, with rigid control of the natural appetites. Shiva's life-positive character embodies wisdom that goes beyond the conventional religious view of things. It is the kind of wisdom that is the foundation of the schools of Indian and Tibetan Tantrism and that also informs the "sexual alchemy" of the later Taoist masters in China.

Both the Tantric masters and the Taoist adepts knew that sexuality in itself is not a hindrance to spiritual maturation. They promoted, on the contrary, the idea that an impotent eunuch stands a slim chance of realizing the supreme potential of spiritual evolution—enlightenment or liberation. Instead of recommending the anxious suppression of the libido, lest it should interfere with the sacred task of spiritual transformation, they favored a sex-positive philosophy. They even designed special practices to utilize this most powerful impulse in us for the process of psychospiritual transmutation. Of course, they did not condone the kind of "sexploitation" that is the liability of the ordinary individual, particularly in our post-sexual-revolution days. Rather, they were interested in the right use of the sexual energy.

In Taoism, the accent lies on a balanced, healthy life through the well-regulated employment of sexuality, by which a person may become sensitive to the spiritual dimension. In Tantrism, the sexual disciplines primarily serve the purpose of self-transcendence to the point of utter bliss. In the former tradition, the "sexual arts" are closely connected with medicine; in the latter tradition they form part of the liberation technology better known as Yoga. Whereas in Taoism sexual intercourse (without male orgasm) is used to manipulate the hormonal system of the body for better health, in Tantrism the focus is principally on the energy exchange between the sex partners. In the Tantric tradition, the male bias is more overt than in the schools of Taoism, though in the latter tradition it is implicit in the prescription to preserve the semen at all costs.

In Hindu Tantrism, where intercourse is linked with the whole notion of sacrifice, the ritual rule against seminal emission is not as absolute as in Buddhist Tantrism. But for both traditions the crux of this sexual ritualism is the same: to restore the body-mind to perfect equilibrium, which coincides with the absolute bliss of enlightenment. The general idea behind these schools of thought is that we are from birth in a state of disequilibrium because of the differentiation of our physical bodies into male and female. This differentiation, known as "dimorphism" in Western physiology, sets up a tension in us. We then seek release from it by trying to merge with the opposite sex, either sexually or emotionally, or both.

Orgasm is the closest simulation of the absolute bliss (*ananda*) that, according to Hindu tradition, we are all unconsciously striving for. But orgasmic pleasure is only a trickle in comparison to that bliss, and it is of course disappointingly ephemeral. The nervous discharge that accompanies orgasm creates a momentary state of balance, but that balance is on a very reduced level of energy.

The Tantric practitioners recognize the error in this popular approach, which seeks self-completion by external means, namely sexual union. They are more interested in heightening the level of psychosomatic energy and in intensifying awareness, until there is the breakthrough into the transcendental dimension of bliss. They engage sexual intercourse as a spiritual discipline rather than for hedonistic reasons.

This entails the insight that every individual is, psychologically speaking, both male and female, and that therefore the desired unitive or balanced state does not occur externally but internally—in consciousness. Thus, for the Tantric practitioner, the outward sexual act is essentially a symbolic ritual of the real work, which is performed in consciousness. Indeed, the "right-hand" (*dakshina*) schools of Tantrism do not even condone actual sexual congress.

However, the left-hand approach (*vama-acara*), which involves sexual intercourse (*maithuna*) with a suitable partner, has the advantage of increasing the level of psychosomatic energy and thus of including the physical dimension in the process of psychospiritual transformation. Actual sexual intercourse involves an energy exchange between the partners in the Tantric ritual, which enhances the unification process that is strived for on the level of consciousness.

At the point of enlightenment, the Tantric practitioner realizes the transcendental unity of Male and Female, Shiva and Shakti. This condition is known as "great delight" (*maha-sukha*), since it cannot be diminished by anything, not even by the act of ejaculation, which typically concludes the male partner's experience of sexual pleasure in ordinary circumstances.

Tantra is the technology of joy on many levels—from sexual

pleasure to transcendental bliss. It is a yogic art that explores the hidden dimensions of the unity of body and mind, which modern science is only now beginning to acknowledge. It reminds us that our guilt about sex is only an added complication that we superimpose on our false relationship to sexual pleasure. Instead of viewing sex as a means of higher human growth, we tend to use it as a fleeting consolation or a way of asserting power and dominance over another. Perhaps our guilt feelings are not so much about engaging our "lower" functions as about not finding the bliss of transcendental consciousness.

Tantrism, or Tantra, challenges us to a radically different view about ourselves and sexuality: to view sex as a lawful, if limited, expression of our innate bliss, and at the same time as a means of getting in touch with that unalloyed delight that is the very nature of reality. According to Tantra, the body is the temple of the divine or transcendental reality. But for this to be *functionally* true of us, and not merely in principle true, we must discover and live from the point of view of that great delight. Then everything, including our sexuality, will be transformed. Our lives become creative play (*lila*).

21

THE JEWEL IN THE LOTUS:
SACRAMENTAL SEXUALITY

Ever since the pioneering sexological works of Van de Velde (the Benjamin Spock of married folk), we have had no dearth of sex books, filled with good advice, prescriptions for successful love-making, and complete with graphic illustrations. For the connoisseur there are also illustrated translations of such exotic Oriental works as the *Kama-Sutra*, the *Ananga-Ranga,* and *The Playful Variations of Master Tung.* We can learn from them a sophisticated technology of sexual positions and other means of maximizing one's own pleasure and that of one's partner. These popular "pillow books" may help us overcome inhibitions and personal limitations. However, they do not particularly advocate the viewpoint of *sex as a sacred activity or sacrament.* Their focus is on bodily pleasure, not on spiritual bliss and self-transcendence.

To learn about the arcane art of sacred sexuality, we must turn to the rather esoteric literature of Taoism and especially Tantrism. Taoism is the Chinese quietistic tradition going back to the *Tao Te Ching* ascribed to the legendary Lao Tzu ("Elder"). It revolves around the concept of the *tao* ("way"), the nameless immortal Reality.

The later Taoist writings contain a great deal of sexological information. A classic work is *The Tao of Sex* by Howard S. Levy and Akira Ishihara, which is a translation of the sexological materials in the tenth-century Japanese medical encyclopedia called *Ishimpo.*[1] Other Taoist scriptures are more concerned with the circulation of energy and the sublimation process. Here the modern interpretations of Mantak Chia and Stephen T. Chang contain the most competent and helpful practical information.[2]

By comparison, the scriptures of Tantrism, written in Sanskrit and known as Tantras, tend to be far less accessible. Although still only inadequately researched, these works have found competent interpreters in Sir John Woodroffe (alias Arthur Avalon) and Manoranjan Basu.[3] Tantrism is the broad religious and philosophical tradition focusing on the feminine cosmic principle, or *shakti*. The word *tantra* means "loom" or "web" and is esoterically explained as "that which expands wisdom (*jnana*)."

The *shakti* is the central agency for that expansion of gnosis. The Yoga associated with Tantrism is *kundalini-yoga*, the *kundalini* being a form of the universal *shakti*. This divine force is located in a potential state at the base of the spine. By awakening it and conducting it to the "thousand-petaled lotus" at the crown of the head, the Tantric aspirant (*sadhaka*) is graced with temporary ecstatic self-transcendence. In the state of "transconceptual ecstasy" (*nirvikalpa-samadhi*), the practitioner tastes the bliss of the Absolute (*brahman*). The principal means of accomplishing this ascent of the *shakti* in the body are concentration (visualization) and breath control.

Both the Taoist and the Tantric works contain a host of practical details about the art of sexual love. They encourage our sexual creativity and our natural interest in magnifying the delight between ourselves and our lovers. They also strongly advocate an erotic technology that is intended to give practitioners a tangible experience of the sacred, be it called *brahman* or *tao*.

What can we learn from Taoism and Tantrism for our own spiritually integrated practice of sex? First of all, we need *not* become full-fledged Taoists or Tantrics to benefit from the insights of these esoteric traditions. All we need to do is to approach them with a receptive mind and an open heart and with the desire to bring all aspects of our lives, including our sexuality, into alignment with the Divine.

Sexual intercourse, even at its most ordinary, is more than skin impinging on skin. It is a form of communication. No words need be exchanged for this to be true. We communicate ourselves in our sexual embrace: our love or lust and our peace or anxiety. Unless our partner is a particularly insensitive individual, our message always comes across, though sometimes on a subliminal level only.

The reason for this effectiveness of communication is that sexual intercourse is an intense form of energy exchange between individuals. That is why sometimes we feel charged by our partner and sometimes we feel drained. Sometimes sex is not only exciting but uplifting, and sometimes it is a letdown. Sacred sexuality is the art and discipline of turning love-making into whole-body loving, of experiencing ourselves and our partner against the eternal backdrop of unconditional love (*prema*) or bliss (*ananda*) of the ultimate Reality.

Obviously, before we can practice sacred sexuality, we must first become sensitive to psychophysical energy (known as *prana* in Sanskrit and *chi* in Chinese). *Hatha-yoga, tai chi*, or simply conscious breathing can help us become more aware of the flow of energy in our body-mind and its energy connection to the environment. The regular use of biocircuits ("Eeman screens") can also greatly facilitate that sensitivity.[4] So long as we look upon our partner as a "meat body," we are apt to treat him or her as a means to an end—a tool for gratifying our own pleasure.

Sacred sexuality, by contrast, presupposes that we are capable of seeing ourselves and our partner in the light of the Divine. It presupposes that we are able to encounter the spiritual Reality, or transcendental Self, in our sexual relationship and play. Only then can we go beyond the anxious pursuit of orgasm. We must bring to our sexual relationship a measure of self-transcendence (surrender) and relaxation of the need to be merely pleasurized.

We should not become neurotic about orgasm—either having it or not having it. Rather, we should relax our concern about it and instead find the delight that comes with being simply present and in heartfelt relationship with one another. This also entails that we should not indulge in erotic fantasies about our partner but actually *see* him or her. Without seeing or experiencing our partner as he or she is, we cannot be drawn into the great Mystery that lies beyond the masks we habitually wear in order to defend ourselves. Fantasies prevent us from being real and present in the moment. They block out the Mystery of life and exclude us from its innate bliss.

Sacred sexuality is a meditative occasion. Hence we should prepare for it as we would for meditation. This includes, for instance, consecrating one's bedroom by tidying it and, perhaps, burning incense and decorating it with flowers. We should also arrange to be undisturbed for a few hours. Some couples keep their bedroom very tidy, clean, and "conscious" at all times, which is preferable. "Pros" decorate it with spiritual art, reminding them of the spiritual purpose of sex—Tibetan *thankas*, paintings, posters, sculptures, gongs. Or they have a picture of their teacher prominently displayed. Some couples develop their own elaborate ritual, complete with the recitation of potent sounds (*mantra*), the drawing of mystic diagrams (*yantra*), and similar yogic ceremonial aids. Others like to keep it very simple.

What is most important, however, is always to bring the right attitude to the occasion. Whether we are in a mood of sobriety or gaiety, we should always remain aware of the sacredness of the sexual play. Obviously, it is advisable to engage sex only when we feel well, balanced, and positive and to abstain when we are sick, agitated, collapsed, or needy. In other words, we should approach the sexual occasion as much as possible in a condition of wholeness, rather than expect to be made whole or to be consoled or fulfilled by it. Then sacred sex will help integrate our being on a deeper level.

Part of preparing our personal environment for the sacred occasion is that we cleanse our body and mind. To shake off the concerns of the day we would do well to relax or sit in meditation for a while, preceded by a shower or bath and followed, perhaps, by a gentle mutual massage.

The actual sexual play is entirely a matter of personal style and preference. Whether we are active/performative or more passive/contemplative, our attention should be on being present here and now, feeling our body-mind and that of our partner and cultivating the great eloquent Silence as it is expanding in us.

In Tantrism, the woman generally sits in the man's lap, which means that she is in control of all movement. Taoism permits a great variety of postures. It also recommends all kinds of fairly technical tricks for intensifying the build-up of nervous energy during sex play. In the last analysis, however, it is not so important what we do. What matters is *how* we do what we do. It is our inner disposition that is critical. This cannot be emphasized enough.

Clearly, the right attitude to sacred sex cannot be cultivated in isolation from our behavior during the rest of the day. We cannot hope to embrace our partner with love and reverence at night but treat her or him as a casual sex object during the day. The success of our sexual discipline depends on our attitude to life as a whole. We cannot compartmentalize our existence without damaging our psyche and relationships.

For the duration of sacred sex (called *maithuna* in Sanskrit), the Tantric partners look upon each other as God and Goddess. Their awareness of each other is transplanted from the material level to the domain of energy and beyond. For most of us who have very little background in visualization and religious mythology, this will not be possible at first or as a rule. However, we can all develop the ability to approach our sexual partner with reverence and clarity and in a mood of love and surrender.

Gradually we will be able to see more in him or her than the individual who is so familiar to us. In fact, we will find that he or she becomes less and less familiar and more and more part of the great Mystery, which is our own hidden essence.

Deep and conscious breathing is the principal means of remaining sensitive to the energy dimension during sexual intercourse. This practice is especially important when we approach orgasm. It permits us to distribute the built-up preorgasmic energy throughout our body, thus preventing orgasm which generally ends the sacred energy play. If, however, orgasm occurs we should simply remain present in our sensory awareness and also in our love-communion, using the breath to guide the mounting sensation to the body as a whole (rather than merely to the genitals) and, beyond the body, to our partner and the cosmos.

It is important not to disengage physical contact abruptly. Intercourse is an intense mingling of our energies, particularly when it is combined with conscious discipline. If orgasm is avoided, our body will remain highly charged after intercourse. It is unwise to manipulate our nervous system to the point of near-orgasm if we cannot live with the resulting charge afterward, without becoming frustrated. Again, breathing can be very useful in diffusing possible tension resulting from overstimulation without orgasmic discharge.

Couples interested in sacred sex must be willing to experiment and make mistakes. This is not a path for the meek, the weak, or the indiscriminate. It is very easy to delude oneself, notably in the spiritual arena. Therefore it is always good to remember that, at least according to Tantrism, the ultimate form of sexual congress does not involve any sexual excitation whatsoever. The couple experience themselves as male God (Shiva) and Goddess (Shakti), absorbed in bliss rather than orgasm.

Thus, the Tantric *yogin* or *yogini* sacrifices orgasm for the great bliss of self-forgetfulness. Western practitioners of the art of sacred sexuality should, however, be wary of pursuing that bliss as they might pursue a pet idea or favored activity. It escapes us even as we make it our goal because it is ever present. Our primary obligation is, therefore, to be present and to discover that bliss in every moment, whether we are engaging in sex or not.

Sacred sex is simply a temporary intensification of our general commitment to a self-transcending life. Sex is never our salvation. It is only another, if powerful, opportunity to realize the great Tantric truth that we are presently free and inherently blissful.

NOTES

1. See H.S. Levy and A. Ishihara, *The Tao of Sex* (Lower Lake, CA: Integral Publishing, 1989).

2. See Mantak Chia and Maneewan Chia, *Healing Love Through the Tao: Cultivating Female Sexual Energy* (Huntington, NY: Healing Tao Books, 1986) and Mantak Chia with Michael Winn, *Taoist Secrets of Love: Cultivating Male Sexual Energy* (Santa Fe, NM: Aurora Press, 1984); Stephen T. Chang, *The Tao of Sexology: The Book of Infinite Wisdom* (San Francisco: Tao Publishing, 1986).

3. See Arthur Avalon (J. Woodroffe), *Tantra of the Great Liberation (Mahanirvana Tantra)* (New York: Dover Publications, repr. 1972) and Shakti and Shakta (New York: Dover Publications, repr. 1978). See also M. Basu, *Fundamentals of the Philosophy of Tantras* (Calcutta: Mira Basu Publishers, 1986).

4. An Eeman screen is a device for enhancing and balancing the energy flow in the body. It is typically constructed of copper mesh or plate to which a wire is attached. One screen is placed under the pelvis, with the wire being held in the right hand, a second screen is placed under the head, with the wire being held in the left hand.

22

IS NONHARMING (AHIMSA)
AN OLD-FASHIONED VALUE?

Homo homini lupus, "Man is a wolf among men." Freud, who quoted this Latin saying, remarked gloomily: "Who has the courage to dispute it in the face of all the evidence?" An array of psychologists, sociologists, and philosophers have reiterated the same view, arguing that aggression is innate to human beings.

But if aggression is innate to us, so is gentleness and the ability to go beyond our murderous instincts. Only an utter pessimist would deny that it is possible for us to live in peace and harmony with our fellow beings and Nature at large. We do not *need* to murder a hundred million people by warfare and torture, as we have done in this century alone. We are free to follow a different course of action. We can cultivate nonviolence, or nonharming, as a viable lifestyle.

Nor is this a mere utopian ideal. Here and there in past eras, and even in our own times, men and women have succeeded in living together cooperatively, without war and strife. Some monastic communities have achieved this great ideal at least during part of their history. Village communities in sheltered environs, which are too remote for curious tourists, are still achieving it today. It is done not for any metaphysical reasons, but simply because everyone's survival depends on the spirit of cooperation.

However, at a particular level in a person's spiritual development, nonviolence becomes something more than an economic or social exigency. It becomes an expression of the inner feeling of unity with everything.

Nonaggressiveness, or nonharming, has been hailed as a cardinal virtue in all major religious traditions of the world. Thus, it has for centuries been central to Yoga. In Patanjali's two-thousand-year-old *Yoga-Sutra*, nonharming (*ahimsa*) is introduced as one of the five practices constituting the "great vow" of the moral disciplines (*yama*).

What does the virtue of nonharming mean to the contemporary Western Yoga student? Is *ahimsa* merely a romantic ideal? Or is it, as Patanjali insists, universally and unconditionally valid? Is this still plausible in our far more complex world? In our century it was Mahatma Gandhi, a master of *karma-yoga* (the path of self-transcending action), who held up high the ancient ideal of *ahimsa*. He also demonstrated its political effectiveness through his stance of passive resistance. Gandhi inspired the modern philosophy and practice of nonviolent social action through demonstrations, sit-ins, teach-ins, petitioning, fasting, and so on. Nonviolent campaigns of social reform have been surprisingly successful, bearing witness to the transformative power of nonharming.

The answer to the question posed above must be: *Ahimsa* is as relevant today as it was at the time of Patanjali and of Gautama the Buddha, another stalwart spokesman for nonviolence. What we need to examine is *how* we can translate the ideal of nonharming into daily practice—for ourselves, our local community, and our global society.

Members of some Jaina sects in India wear a mask to filter the air, lest they should unwittingly inhale and take the life of small creatures. This is a religious custom that few of us would want to follow. Nevertheless, upon closer inspection this extreme practice contains a useful lesson: Our life is built on the sacrificial death of others. We are involuntarily murdering creatures with every breath—a massacre that not even a mask can prevent. For, we constantly annihilate billions of invisible microbes so that we may live. We ourselves are a link in the great food chain of life, destined to die and be food for microbic creatures.

We need not stop breathing or feeding ourselves, or constantly "turn the other cheek," but we must appreciate how we owe our life to other beings and how they owe their lives to us. When we truly see this vast interconnectedness, it becomes easy for us to cultivate an attitude of reverence for life, which is essentially an attitude of nonharming and of ego-transcending love.

We must train our sensitivity to the fact that we are not alone in the universe but are interdependent cells of a cosmic body. Spiritual life is largely a matter of taking responsibility for the things we have understood about ourselves and the world we live in. This includes assuming responsibility for our destructive aggression, as it reveals itself to us in ever subtler forms.

As Patanjali states, nonharming must be practiced under all conditions, which means in thought, word, and deed. Our self-inspection can begin with our active life. For instance, we may ask ourselves whether our livelihood involves harming others in ways that are not morally justifiable. As a writer and publisher I have become progressively aware of the fact that I am co-responsible for the destruction of forests, which are the habitat of countless species, not least human tribal groups. I have begun to take remedial actions, such as using recycled and acid-free paper that will last longer, reusing envelopes and other paper rather than discarding them, and so on. I know that I can and should do more.

Another important area of self-inspection concerns our social relationships—our family life, friendships, and business relationships. How are we destructively aggressive in them? Where could we begin to practice *ahimsa* more seriously? How do we typically express our unlove and lack of compassion or empathy?

One way of going about this is to ask our relatives and friends to give us their undoubtedly painful feedback. We may find that we tend to come across as overly aggressive, cold, or unapproachable. We may be told that we don't let others express themselves, or that we are poor listeners. There are numerous ways in which we can practice unlove, just as there are countless ways in which we can be loving and compassionate.

We can cause harm not only by our physical actions but also by our speech. Words spoken in anger or out of inconsiderateness may hurt others as much as or more than a slap in the face. Another area of psychological harming is our competitiveness when it becomes callous. We try to outstrip each other and in the process strip ourselves and others of all dignity.

Then there is the whole matter of how we maintain our body's energies and health. Unless we are strict vegetarians, we consume meat, fish, eggs, and dairy products. Quite apart from any religious considerations, we must be concerned about the fact that our dietary habits are locked into a vast industry that is not known for its moral scruples. The meals we eat tend to come from factory-farmed animals that are widely treated with unbelievable cruelty ("because animals don't feel pain as we do"). Cows are kept artificially pregnant to yield milk, while their calves are deprived of motherly affection, forced to eat a monotonous milk-replacing diet to ensure that their flesh will be as white as the market demands; chickens are debeaked and cooped up in torturously small cages; pigs are tail-docked and kept in miniscule pens in the dark, forced to eat from sheer boredom, doing nothing but waiting to be slaughtered in an often brutal way.

Thus our food habits endorse an industry, running to some fifty billion dollars a year, that blatantly violates the ideal of nonharming. It also contributes in a major way to the massive degradation of the environment. Our medical needs and choices have a similarly tragic effect, for they support the often gruesome exploitation of animals in laboratories.

Similarly, our hunger for entertainment leads to animal abuse in a variety of ways—from hunting to rodeos and races to seemingly innocuous zoos and circuses. Much could also be said about how our conspicuous consumption directly or indirectly disadvantages other nations, causing hunger and plight to millions of fellow-humans.

All our actions have moral repercussions. For instance, doing our duty as an upright citizen involves paying taxes every year. But our taxes help support a vast military industry that revolves around violence, and which in effect leads to countless deaths and untold pain around the world. It would be foolish to withhold taxes, but we can work for a long-overdue tax reform and, more importantly, protest against the ways in which our tax money is spent.

Finally, the ideal of nonharming is not confined to physical or verbal expression. Our very thoughts are powerful. They determine the subtle ways in which we relate to life, especially how we interact with others. If we are down, we tend to drag our environment down. If we are emotionally buoyant, our happiness uplifts those around us. Even if we do not mean to harm another person, our coldness or indifference is a form of harming. Whenever we are not present *as* love, we inevitably reduce our own life and the life in others. Hence we are responsible for *how* we are present in the world, even when we are on our own, because our field is interconnected with the fields of everyone and everything else.

Ahimsa, as a manifestation of self-transcending love, is a building block of spiritual practice. Genuine Yoga is impossible without it. Nonharming is certainly *not* an old-fashioned value.

23

THE PRACTICE OF ECO-YOGA

All life is interconnected and ultimately interdependent. This is the subject-matter of ecology. Very simply, ecology is the study of the vital relationships between plants and animals (or humans) and the environment in which they live. Often the word is used to refer to the living being/environment connection itself.

Our planet has been likened to a gigantic spaceship whose resources are limited. While it is true that the Earth's resources are by no means inexhaustible, a far more important fact is that our home planet is vastly more complex than any technological device could ever be. It is, as biologist James Gordon Lovelock reminded our generation, a living organism, which he called "Gaia." As a living organism, the Earth is a finely balanced system of forces.

Over the past several decades, this equilibrium has been seriously disturbed by unecological patterns of life characteristic mainly of the "civilized" countries of the world, leading to what is called the "ecological crisis." Many factors are involved in this very serious crisis, notably overpopulation, disadvantageous population distribution (e.g., huge metropolitan areas), overconsumption, wasteful patterns of consumption, inappropriate use of technology, and not least egocentric, shortsighted ways of thought.

What does all this have to do with Yoga? *Everything*. Yoga is intrinsically ecological. All Yoga is what I call "Eco-Yoga." As the *Bhagavad-Gita* (II.48), the oldest Yoga scripture, puts it, Yoga is balance (*samatva*). We need not understand this in purely psychological terms. When we are inwardly balanced, we are also balanced in relationship to our environment. This is borne out by the comprehensive and rigorous ethical code of Yoga, which covers the whole range of the Yoga practitioner's relationship to the environment and other living beings.

This code is expressed in the five rules of moral restraint (*yama*). Thus, nonharming (*ahimsa*) consists in reverence for all forms of life. This implies, for instance, that we should choose a lifestyle that will not rob other creatures of their ecological niches. Also, if we take this rule seriously, we must adopt a vegetarian diet. Failing this, we should ensure that our consumption of animal products (meat, eggs, and dairy products) at least does not in any way support the cruel practice of factory-farming of animals.

The yogic rule of nonstealing (*asteya*) implies, for example, that we should not take more than we need for the upkeep of our body-mind. Few of us are willing to live in the Spartan fashion to which *yogins* are accustomed. However, there are many things we can do to adapt to this moral obligation. Thus, we can avoid what has been called "conspicuous consumption," including the needless wasting of food. Instead, we could learn to use our surplus (which is often simply destined to become garbage) to improve the living conditions of our less fortunate fellow humans.

Similarly, the moral rule of greedlessness (*aparigraha*) is understood as a comprehensive demand to relate to life in a balanced, nongrasping manner, which respects the right of others to share the resources of our planet. Conscious living is a balance between giving and taking. So, for instance, when we have to cut down a tree on our property, we should plant at least one new tree. Eco-yogic thinking demands that we help replenish our planet's resources.

The yogic call for purity (*shauca*), which is a part of the rules of self-discipline (*niyama*), can also be understood in a wider ecological sense. We should do our utmost to eliminate pollution in our own life and to support those efforts that seek to clean up our environment at large.

"Eco-Yoga" is my way of describing the now necessary convergence between traditional yogic spirituality and social activism focusing on ecological concerns. I intuit that in the final decade of this century we will face an increasing environmental crisis affecting all our lives deeply. We cannot afford any longer to exclusively pursue quietistic goals. We must also take responsibility for the environment in which we live, and that means to recover our sense of the sacredness of this planet and to actively participate in its ecological recovery.

Metaphysically speaking, the challenge confronting us is to learn to respect both transcendence *and* immanence. To put it concretely, we cannot hope to find ourselves, never mind the Divine, so long as we obstruct our view by piling up mountains of garbage or by opaqueing the air with toxic pollutants. Instead, we must learn to cooperate with Nature, which is the very basis for any spiritual effort we wish to make. We must be willing to be loyal not only to our chosen spiritual path but also to our habitat.

The tradition of Tantrism has hailed the body as a most valuable instrument for realizing the Divine, or Reality. We must similarly recognize the immense value of our planet. The Earth is our body, and it is the only one we have. If we destroy it, we commit suicide.

Here are some guidelines for cultivating the eco-yogic process:

1. Make a serious attempt at understanding our present age and the historical forces shaping it. Since we live in a complex pluralistic civilization, our lives are inevitably subject to all kinds of sociocultural currents, which we need to understand in order to cultivate our own authenticity. In particular, we need to clearly comprehend the magnitude of the ecological crisis humanity is facing today.

2. Become fully aware of, and informed about, the problem. Study books like Paul and Anne Ehrlich's *The Population Bomb* (1968) and *The Population Explosion* (1990); Barbara Ward's *The Home of Man* (1976); Thomas Berry's *The Dream of the Earth* (1988); Duane Elgin's *Voluntary Simplicity* (1981); Mihajlo Mesarovic's and Eduard Pestel's Club-of-Rome report *Mankind at the Turning Point* (1974); Jonathan Porritt's *Seeing Green* (1984); Lester Brown's ongoing *State of the World* reports; the Sierra Club's *Ecotactics* (1970) edited by John G. Mitchell and Constance L. Stallings; *The Greenhouse Trap* (1990) edited by Francesca Lyman *et al*. All these publications, and many other good books, contain a wealth of valuable information that has immediate relevance. But there are a few books that can be particularly recommended as practical manuals: *The*

Global Ecology Handbook: What You Can Do About the Environmental Crisis (1990) edited by Walter H. Corson; *50 Simple Things You Can Do To Save the Earth* (1989), *50 Simple Things Kids Can Do To Save the Earth* (1990), and *The Recycler's Handbook* (1990) by the EarthWorks Group in Berkeley, California; and *The Simple Act of Planting a Tree* (1990) by Treepeople with Andy and Katie Lipkis, published by J.P. Tarcher in Los Angeles.

You don't have to become an expert, but you ought to know what is happening around you that affects you and the life of your children.

3. Live a simpler, ecologically sensitive life. Take stock of your consumption patterns and decide how you can help reduce energy consumption and pollution in your own immediate environment. For instance, ask yourself: Do I need to have so many lights on? Do I really need to run the air conditioner or heater, or could I insulate my house better and thus cut down energy wastage? Do I need to use the car quite so often, or could I plan my trips more wisely and perhaps use car pools? Do I need to flush the toilet with every use, or have fifteen-minute showers every day? Why couldn't I recycle cans and bottles? Can I really not afford to buy healthier organic food? Am I simply too lethargic to use vegetable waste to make a compost heap in the garden? And so on. Big change begins by doing the "little" things — *now.*

4. Join forces with a local ecology group and become politically active. Yoga is not merely inwardness. Nor are Yoga and political commitment incompatible. All too often Yoga practitioners are concerned with their own salvation, ignoring the larger context in which they live. In the final analysis, this is not only selfish and contrary to the spirit of Yoga but also counterproductive. For the environment impinges on us. How can you, for example, hope to cultivate breath control in a polluted neighborhood? Or how can you hope to maintain a healthy body-mind when the soil on which your food grows is poisoned by chemicals? Or how can you hope to achieve the necessary inner stillness for meditation and prayer to transform your psyche when your eardrums vibrate from the constant cacophony on the streets and in the sky?

At the very least, support activist groups like Greenpeace, Friends of the Earth, Sierra Club, National Wildlife Federation, or the Elmwood Institute.

5. Cultivate self-understanding by scrutinizing the motives behind your spiritual odyssey, and be willing to recognize and work with neurotic tendencies masquerading as spiritual ideals. Don't necessarily trust your own self-image, but consult benevolent others who may serve you as more accurate mirrors of your own character. Inadequate self-understanding frequently leads to wrong action.

6. Study the spiritual traditions of the world to deepen your understanding of your preferred path. This will help you appreciate the complementarity of the Earth's religious and spiritual traditions. It will also reduce the tendency toward parochialism, cultism, spiritual elitism, and other forms of exclusivism. Such study can help you cultivate the admirable and indeed essential virtues of compassion and tolerance, which facilitate cooperation and ecological living.

7. Stay in touch with your natural environment. Living in cities seduces people into having a merely abstract relationship to the Earth. It is important to touch the soil, tend flowers or trees, taste clean spring water, see the exuberance of wildlife, and so forth. Inwardness without such grounding is often little more than neurotic escape. Wholeness requires the transformative touch of the Earth as well as the blessing from the "heaven within."

8. Daily remind yourself that life is a precious gift, which must not be squandered, neglected, or abused. If your heart is open, gratitude and praise will flow easily from your lips. Our Western upbringing, generally speaking, does not make us predisposed to express our gratitude (or our other emotions), and it teaches us to be critical rather than full of praise. There is, of course, no need to withhold criticism where it is due, but it is often received more readily when it is tempered with compassion and praise (which can be viewed as an active form of compassion).

Living in our postmodern world has wounded us all in one way or another, and there is much need for healing. Praise and the expression of gratitude are, in my experience, excellent means of soothing our pain (*duhkha*) and restoring hope. When we experience life as a spiritual opportunity for which we are grateful, the world ceases to be our enemy. We will still share in the harvest of our collective karma and feel sorrow at the exploitation of the Earth, but we will also begin to feel a deeper affinity for everyone and everything—which is healing in itself. We become true citizens of the ecosystem, consciously casting our vote for its future in the way we live each moment.

24

DIE WHILE YOU LIVE: LAST-HOUR YOGA

There is an oft-quoted verse in the *Bhagavad-Gita* (VIII.6) that is widely understood as declaring that a person's last thought on the death-bed determines his or her post-mortem destiny. In Juan Mascaro's popular translation, the stanza in question reads as follows:

> For on whomsoever one thinks at the last moment of life, unto him in truth he goes, through sympathy with his nature.

On first hearing, this sounds as if death furnishes us with a magic wand by which we can transmogrify ourselves into absolutely anything that captures our imagination when we draw the last breath. And this is how popular Indian tradition has caricatured the God-man Krishna's utterance. In the following I will attempt to show that Krishna's teaching is less comical but far more subtle and demanding.

To begin with, we must note that if indeed the more facile interpretation were correct, we would have to discard one of the fundamental principles of Krishna's metaphysics, namely the idea that the cosmos is a process guided by an immutable moral law. It would be perfectly feasible to picture, for example, the following extreme case: A mass murderer who, until the penultimate moment of his life, pursues his ugly trade and then, cunning as he is, spends his very last instant of embodiment thinking about the Absolute. In keeping with the simplistic exegesis of Krishna's word, the murderer would most certainly become instantly coessential with the ultimate Reality. His string of heinous crimes would be forgiven and forgotten in an instant, and he would be rewarded with unexcelled bliss. This possibility rightly offends our sense of justice.

Let us frame another extreme case: A saint who, until the penultimate moment of his life, has not once transgressed the moral laws of the universe, dies in a car accident and his very last thought is one of compassion for the unfortunate driver—the mass murderer in our example—who is also killed. In terms of the popular interpretation, the saint's fate is definitely sealed. He would take a very steep fall from the heights of spiritual attainment to which he had ascended through life-long struggle.

It seems improbable that Krishna should have taught such an outrageous doctrine, which would make nonsense of his whole ethical teaching, the path of Yoga, and the orderliness of creation. So, what did Krishna really say all those many centuries ago? A more literal rendering than Juan Mascaro's widely read paraphrase provides important clues:

> Whatever state-of-existence (*bhava*) he remembers when at last he sheds the body, even that [state-of-existence] does he attain, O son-of-Kunti, always forced-to-become that state-of-existence.

First of all, we find that the enlightened adept Krishna does not speak, as the above-quoted translator would have it, of "someone" upon whom one should fix one's mind, but of a "state-of-existence" (*bhava*). Furthermore, there is a world of difference between "thinking" about something and "remembering" it, which is Krishna's well-chosen term.

Now, "state-of-existence" is not just anything. Rather, the word denotes a whole *category* of existential possibilities within the immeasurable Body Divine. In the most radical sense there are only two major *bhavas* or levels of being: the mutable (*kshara*) or impermanent realm and the immutable (*akshara-bhava*).

From our human perspective, the first level is of course the space-time universe which is the familiar arena of our conditioned experiencing. But the world as we know it is but the outer shell of a vastly more grandiose structure of hierarchically interlocking levels of being. At the apex of it all, pervading and upholding the entire creation, is the Immutable, the Divine.

The *Bhagavad-Gita* distinguishes three more subordinate levels. Closest to the Divine, which is Krishna in his true nature, are the innumerable transcendental Selves called *atman* or *akshara-purusha*. This multitude of eternal Selves forms as it were the cells of the Divine Body. These Selves are also referred to as the Divine

Person's "higher nature" (*para-prakriti*).

When these eternally free Selves are associated with particular body-minds, they become *kshara-purushas* or "perishable selves." These are the many individuals in bondage to the material universe. Ourselves.

The giant body of Nature is really a composite of three cardinal levels of existence. Over and above the material realm there is a vast suprasensible world that is the level of the mind or subtle body. This extends up to the very matrix (*prakriti*) of the objective universe, the playground of the transcendental Selves.

Diagrammatically, this progressive inclusiveness looks as follows:

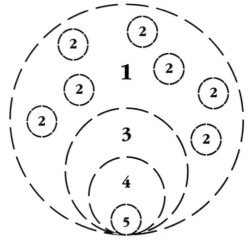

1 = the Whole, Lord Krishna
2 = the countless Selves (*purusha*)
3 = the transcendental ground of the world (*prakriti*)
4 = the suprasensible realm
5 = the material universe

Looked at differently, these various levels are possibilities of "bodily" existence. Depending on which "body," or state-of-existence, we set our heart on, we will obtain that very form of "embodiment" once we have quit our present physical vehicle. Thus we may resume a human form, become an angelic being (*deva*) inhabiting the subtle realm, sink into the cosmic matrix itself as a *prakriti-laya*, or recover our true identity as the Self in the blissful "company" of the Divine Person, Lord Krishna.

The phrase "to set one's heart on something" is perhaps more expressive of the intended meaning of "remembering" than is "thinking." The latter has too abstract a flavor, while the former is indicative of a deep-level process. This becomes clear when one realizes that one of the synonyms of "meditation" is in fact "remembering."

Meditative remembering means sending tap-roots down into the hidden recesses of our being, into the depth-mind (*buddhi*). The depth-mind is the storehouse of the essences of our world-experiencing. It has been likened to a net whose knots are the impressions left behind by our volitional activity.

Meditation is a partial enactment of the process of dying. Conversely, death is the meditative process taken to its logical conclusion. At death, the mind disentangles itself from the physical body, and the center of identity is shifted to the subtle vehicle—the so-called astral body or "subtle vehicle" (*sukshma-sharira*). The quintessence of the contents of the mind, in the form of the subliminal impressions (*samskara*) stored away in the depth-mind, is the factor that determines the after-death fate of the deceased according to the iron-law of moral retribution or karma.

This event is a kind of "remembering," for it is by the power of the depth-mind, the hidden memory, that justice is done to the virtuous and the sinner alike, each according to his or her deeds or, more precisely, volitions. People who have been on the verge of death, or who have been resuscitated after having been clinically dead, often report that they saw their life's journey flash past their inner eye.

We can easily imagine what this remembering on the threshold of death would consist of in the case of an ordinary man. He would be presented with fleeting scenes from his childhood, his adolescence, his love affairs, marriages, career, and leisure activities, his role as a parent, friend, and colleague. He would momentarily re-live all the joyous and sad moments of his life and understand their deep purpose. He would recognize an overall pattern that is the essential structure informing his mode of existence in the hereafter and his eventual rebirth.

Self-transcending spiritual practitioners will undoubtedly have many of the above experiences in common with worldly individuals. But they will look back upon fewer missed opportunities for self-improvement and inner growth. In their depth-mind there will be powerful impressions that are incompatible with re-embodiment in the material realm. If they are advanced, these subliminal activators will outweigh all others.

Individuals who have always lived typical human lives invite rebirth as typical human beings. But those Yoga practitioners who model their whole existence not on mere human standards but on the ultimate Reality will, if they have succeeded in setting up incisive enough impressions in their depth-memory, merge with that Reality.

And if these practitioners are sufficiently advanced on the spiritual path, they will be able to monitor the process of dying and so ensure that no vestiges remain in their depth-mind, which would force them to assume another physical body. In fact, the conscious departure from this world is one of the sure marks by which one can recognize a genuine *yogin* or *yogini*. The Self-realized adept regards the body like a vessel that is engulfed by space, both within and without, the space being the omnipresent Reality.

Death does not shake the adept in the least. Many moving stories are told by disciples who have witnessed their *guru*'s exit from the world—"with a single breath" and a smile. A dying *yogin* in agony or a state of stupor is almost a contradiction in terms. The maxim holds: Show me how you die, and I show you who you are.

But, the reader may ask, what if the Yoga adept drowns unexpectedly or is killed by a stray bullet? Will the element of surprise not outwit him or her? The traditional answer is a most emphatic No. There can be no surprise for the enlightened being—hence the smile. This would imply that the universe is ruled by chance, which is an assumption that is explicitly rejected by the Yoga masters.

In whichever way the masters of Yoga take leave from this world—and, as the poet knew, death has ten thousand doors—they will have foreknowledge of their death. There are too many well-attested examples for this to be purely fictional icing on the cake of hagiolatry. How such knowledge is obtained remains a mystery that need not concern us here.

The process of conscious exit from the body, however, is not a secret—at least not in principle. The archaic *Chandogya-Upanishad* (VIII.6.5–6) discloses the following:

Now, when he thus departs from this body,
then he ascends upward with these rays [of
the sun]. Pronouncing [the sacred syllable]
om, he dies. As soon as the mind is cast off,
he goes to the sun. This, verily, is the
"world door," an entry for the knowers,
[but] a blockage for the ignorant.

On this [there is the following] verse:

There are a hundred and one channels of the heart.
One of these runs to [the crown of] the head.
Going up by it, one reaches immortality.
The others are for departing to various [lower
levels of being]; [they] are for departing to
various [lower levels].

In conscious dying, attention is focused on the axial current of the body, or what is known as the *sushumna-nadi*. This is the only pathway of the life-force (*prana*) that extends from the lowest psychosomatic center (at the base of the spine) to the crown of the head, which is the location of the thousand-petaled lotus, the seat of the mystical sun. This intense focusing of the mind and the life-force within the central channel, and especially on its upper terminal in the head, coincides with the condition of ecstasy (*samadhi*). Then, as the author of the *Hatha-Yoga-Pradipika* (IV.17) observes, time stands still.

Such knowledge is implied in the words of the God-man Krishna who, in the *Bhagavad-Gita* (VIII.5ff), admonishes his would-be follower thus:

He who goes hence at the "end time," abandoning
the body and remembering Me alone—he reaches
My state-of-existence. (5)

He who remembers the Ancient Bard, Governor
[of all the world], smaller than the small,
Supporter of all, of inconceivable form,
sun-colored [and abiding] beyond darkness (6)

—that [*yogin*], at the time of going-forth,
with unmoving mind, yoked by love and by the
power of Yoga, directing the life-force to
[the spot in] the middle of the eye-brow,
comes to that supreme Divine Being (*purusha*). (7)

The first verse of this passage includes a term that invites closer inspection. This is the Sanskrit word *anta-kala*, which I have rendered literally as "end time." A more conventional translation would be "last hour," but "end time" has more instructive connotations.

For the term *anta-kala* is also used in regard to the final dissolution of creation during the onset of a cosmic "night," when the Creator is asleep and when all manifestation is resolved into a state of latency. By extension, *anta-kala* can also be applied to the segments of the flux of events—those spells of creative respite of the world process that cause the pulse of life. Time, we know, is discontinuous. This modern insight has long been anticipated by the Yoga masters of yore who talked of time-quanta (*kshana*) which alone are imbued with reality, whereas time itself is but a mental construct.

What does this have to do with our main theme? If time is merely a series of infinitesimally small "instants," which are perceptible only to the *yogin*, then we must conclude that we die and are reborn in rapid succession.

Life and death, in this view, are intimately and inseparably linked. If we now transfer Krishna's ethical imperative that we should remember him at the "end time" to this situation, we arrive at a remarkable insight: We must remember the Divine Person not only when the Reaper knocks on our door, but in every moment of our life.

Students of the *Bhagavad-Gita* know that this is precisely what Lord Krishna expects from his devotees. The vocation of the practitioner of Yoga is a full-time occupation. Only thus can he or she hope to conquer *kala*—a Sanskrit word that means both "death" and "time."

Death borders upon our birth,
and our cradle stands in the grave.

(*Epistles*, 2)

25

IMMORTALITY AND FREEDOM:
INDIA'S PERSPECTIVE

Nothing can intellectually convince me that we survive physical death. All the empirical evidence that I have examined, and all the evidence that could possibly be marshalled in favor of our postmortem survival cannot change my mind. My *mind*—that is, my sober rational mind, trained extensively in academic skepticism and well exercised in agnosticism.

Luckily, however, my rational mind does not exhaust who I am. I have other cognitive capacities that I can bring into play when pondering my destiny after death. Yet, curiously enough, I remain intellectually unconverted even by my own firsthand experiences of psychospiritual states in which the body-mind, as I normally experience it, is apparently transcended. I believe that my situation is shared by a good many other people, who cultivate doubt as an appropriate professional attitude. They, too, remain rationally unconvinced by the thousands of cases of near-death experiences, out-of-body experiences, and body-transcending mystical raptures.

This is both fortunate and unfortunate. It is unfortunate because in most cases this means that our lives remain relatively closed. It is fortunate because in at least some cases it provokes the kind of curiosity that turns the searchlight of science to matters that are all too frequently dismissed as metaphysical nonsense.

As I said before, reason or intellect is only one aspect of what I know myself to be. It has its place, but when it comes to metaphysical matters I have always employed it rather judiciously, because I understood early on that, generally speaking, its competence lies more in the structuring of information than in the acquisition of knowledge. And so, for the past twenty-five years I have with great personal benefit studied the spiritual traditions of India.

While I find many, if not most, of the metaphysical systems spawned on the Indian peninsula quite inadequate as descriptions of reality, they have never failed to inspire me, precisely because I have never approached them solely with the rational scholarly mind. Thus, the mystical intuitions of the *Rig-Veda,* the *Upanishads,* the Yoga scriptures, or the animated wisdom of the saintly literature of medieval India, or even the works and biographies of modern sages have been almost daily nourishment for me, and for this I am deeply grateful.

But for these often quite "outlandish" teachings to be communicative for me, I have always had to approach them with the kind of openness, or open-heartedness, with which one would approach one's wife or husband or a dear friend. What they teach me about myself, that is, my larger being, is of immeasurable value to me. Their communication has always baffled my mind, and continues to do so, but it has also always enriched that native wisdom that we all possess and that comes to the fore when we discipline the rational mind and prevent it from tyrannizing our grasp of reality. Rational thought has the formidable power of whittling into a million pieces what should be grasped intuitively, as a whole.

In this essay, I want to convey some of the great insights about freedom and immortality to which the Hindu genius has given birth over a period of three millennia, insights which have informed my own thinking and feeling about this perennial subject.

It is thought that at the beginning of philosophy stands curiosity. But curiosity, the need to know, has a deeper, emotional root—our fear of death. Though we may deny this fact, or behave as if it were not true of us, our existence is as limited in time as it is limited in space. We know that, like all things, our life is bound to end, and that we have to leave everything that we now call "me" and "mine" behind. As we see our body-mind gradually succumb to the law of entropy, we become increasingly mindful of this irrefutable fact.

We also turn to philosophy, metaphysics, and theology at times of crisis when our lives are threatened. Moreover, philosophical thought is kindled in us when we suffer from what Colin Wilson

dubbed the "outsider" syndrome: when we feel marginal, dis-
placed—whether socially or in our beliefs. In each case, however, I
suggest that we confront the fact that we are not absolute, infinite,
endless, all-powerful, all-knowing, fulfilled, or perfect—attributes
that we reserve for the supreme being called "God" or "ultimate
Reality."

But allow me to travel back in time to the concluding centuries of
the second millennium B.C. The early Indians had ample occasion
for pondering the meaning and purpose of life. The originators of
the *Vedas*, the earliest Indo-European literature, were outsiders who
had come from the steppes of what is now Russia. They were con-
querors surrounded by enemies. They had been semi-nomadic
cattle breeders, but now they had to learn to cultivate the land and
to live with the dangers of the jungle and of seasonal flooding. Their
central deity was Indra, a god of rainstorms, thunder, and war. They
prayed to him for wealth and to avert calamity as well as to gain
victory over the newly won soil and the native inhabitants.

They worshipped Indra by means of the "intoxicating" *soma*
juice, to such an extent that some readers of the Vedas arrived at the
erroneous conclusion that the Vedic Indians were permanently
drunk, unfortunate victims of *soma* addiction. Indra, of course, was
the soma quaffer par excellence, and the humble worshipper saw
himself or herself as only imitating the great god. The *soma*
draught—whatever it may have been, and R. Gordon Wasson suggested it was the mushroom *Amanita muscaria*—was obviously
potent. It altered their consciousness, and while *soma*-"intoxicated"
they experienced themselves as being in the company of Indra and
even as matching the great deity's splendor.

Some people may wonder whether their experiences were purely
hallucinatory or whether they were genuine mystical elevations. I
feel that most likely both held true of them, just as the LSD-takers of
the 1960s and 1970s experienced a mass of inconsequential fire-
works and, occasionally, genuine spiritual breakthroughs that had a
decidedly positive effect on their lives.

But in contrast to the acid-heads of the modern counterculture,
who grew up in a confused secularized society, the Vedic people
were far more likely to experience the sacred dimension of existence,

so that even their hallucinations were apt to assume great personal and social significance. Pharmacology is not destiny, to coin a phrase. A drug may change a person's perception and self-perception but this does not mean that it will inevitably determine, or even have any impact at all, on how that individual will think and behave after the effects have worn off.

Alcohol is a good example, but even a powerful psychogenic drug such as LSD need not, and demonstrably did not always, lead to significant changes in a person's values or lifestyle. Much depends on what one brings to the drug experience and whether one chooses to integrate it with the rest of one's life.

The Vedic seers and sages, and even simple householders doing their daily *soma* sacrifices, were all steeped in sacred values and religious beliefs, which undoubtedly informed their soma-induced peak experiences.

However, here I am more interested in the philosophical distillate of their *soma* experiences. How did their pharmacological excursions find expression in their thoughts and lives? The simple answer is that far from turning them into incompetent *soma* addicts, the sacred draught sensitized them to the numinous hidden dimensions of the cosmos and their own psyche. They *lived* in a world that we would debunk as mythological fancy. Indra, Agni, Rudra; and Surya were deities that had immediate reality for them. Prayers and ceremonial offerings had effective power, influencing the hidden world and the visible world around them. The breath was not oxygen but all-sustaining life-force (*prana*). And death was not the end of human life but a threshold experience, opening up another realm of existence.

With the possible exception of professional thinkers like the Greek sophists and modern university professors of philosophy, for whom thinking is a livelihood, thoughtful people of all cultures and periods have always been provoked to thought by the contemplation of their own finitude. This is well illustrated in the hymns of the ancient *Vedas*. The *soma*-inspired visions and metaphysical flights of their composers reveal to us a culture that was down-to-earth but not crassly materialistic; even when the Vedic people prayed for more rain, more cattle, or victory over the enemy, they never lost sight of the invisible forces that they felt were influencing or guiding their destiny. They believed in and conversed with deities, ancestral spirits, demons, goblins, elves, and a host of other creatures that have been made homeless by scientific thought.

Above all, they believed that after a long, prosperous, and happy life on Earth they could look forward to a joyous life in the hereafter. They did not doubt in the least that death is merely a transition, not an end. For them, the after-death state was a world where milk and honey flow in abundance, providing that one's earthly life has been just and noble. Evil-doers, however, were promised a plunge into bottomless darkness.

The more sensitive or mature souls, who realized that even the most wonderful life on earth is marred by change and death, translated their desire to escape the clutches of death into a higher spiritual impulse. They prayed and prepared themselves for immortality in the domain beyond even the heavenly paradise, where the average faithful individual is reunited with his or her family and friends. They wanted to share the immortality of the disembodied Gods and Goddesses themselves.

Here we have the seed of the later Hindu notion that the core of the human personality is transcendental and perfectly identical with the very ground of the universe, as formulated in the *Upanishads*. *Aham brahma asmi*, "I am the Absolute." *Tat tvam asi*, "That art thou." *Sarvam idam brahma*, "All this is the Absolute." These are the great utterances of the Upanishadic sages. The transcendental Self (*atman*), which is the subjective core of the human personality, is immortal, deathless. It is coessential with the deepest core, or the highest dimension, of the objective universe, which is known as the *brahman*.

All that can be said about that Absolute is that it exists, is singular, supremely conscious (rather than insentient), and utterly blissful. The Upanishadic sages hence spoke of it as Being-Consciousness-Bliss (*sat-cid-ananda*).

What is the relationship between that transcendental Singularity and the space-time world, which is a theater of subjects and objects? The Hindu sages thought deeply about this question, and came up with different answers, which testifies to their philosophical ingenuity.

The authorities of the earliest *Upanishads* still regarded the world as an emanation of the One Being, though they suggested different versions of this belief.

Later thinkers, notably the eminent propounder of Vedantic nondualism, Shankara (788–820 A.D.), moved toward a more sophisticated point of view, which looks upon the world as a product of spiritual ignorance (*avidya*), without being entirely illusory. Some authorities, like the composer of the tenth-century *Yoga-Vasishtha*, took a still more radical stance, suggesting that the phenomenal world is an outright hallucination, and that only the ultimate Being-Consciousness exists. The same idealist view is shared by some schools of Mahayana Buddhism.

What is important to realize is that these metaphysical formulations were not mere speculation or book knowledge. Primarily they were founded in actual yogic realizations. The *Upanishads* are not so much philosophical discourses as testimonies to the mystical experiences of hundreds of sages and adepts of Yoga. They did not content themselves with mere belief in an afterlife, or pious hopes about future immortality. Their quest was to discover immortality in this very lifetime. Freedom was no slogan for them, nor did it have the narrow political connotations it tends to have today. Freedom meant to be radically free, in spirit.

They hoped to free themselves not from political enslavement or the yoke of economic necessity, but from the chains of their own psychomental conditioning. Whatever circumstances they were confronting, they wanted to stand fearless, even blissful, and quite unconcerned about their past, present, and future. In their quest for freedom and immortality, they explored a great variety of means— severe asceticism (*tapas*), absolute renunciation (*vairagya*), and the more integrated disciplines of meditation and ecstasy, which are at the heart of what came to be known as *yoga.*

This was a breakthrough discovery: that in order to acquire immortality, a person did not have to drop the body, but that perfect spiritual freedom could be attained in the embodied form. The ideal of "living liberation" (*jivan-mukti*) was born, and from then on existed side by side with the earlier ideal of "disembodied liberation" (*videha-mukti*).

In its significance for humanity, that discovery is more important than the invention of the wheel or the invention of agriculture and the domestication of animals. And yet, most of humankind is utterly unaware of it. And so the great adepts and sages of Hinduism and other religio-spiritual traditions continue to be ignored. Why is that discovery so significant? Because, once its implications are fully understood, it frees us from the necessity of the religious quest for a paradisaical life in the hereafter, as well as from the search for fulfillment in the conditional realms of existence.

At the same time, it frees us for a realistic, rather than idealistic, attitude toward life. How so? Actors who take their theatrical roles off stage are in serious psychological trouble. This describes our ordinary condition: We generally forget that our roles as marriage partners, parents, householders, breadwinners, car drivers, taxpayers, good citizens, and so on, do not define us exhaustively. Instead, we tend typically to behave as if those diverse roles were our very living cells, as if we amounted to nothing apart from them. We are burdened by this mistaken notion, and yet do not even know that there is an alternative to it.

However, when we understand that we are not identical with *any* of the roles that we so skillfully animate in the course of our conventional lives, we also no longer suffer the limitations of our multiple and often complex roles. Suddenly we stand in a free relationship to them, able to respond to the social game around us, without being swallowed up or diminished by it. We are our "own man." We achieve autonomy, though not the silent heroic type portrayed so well by John Wayne, which is merely another and quite unlikely social role-identity. Rather, our autonomy is founded in our recognition of the primacy of the immortal Consciousness (*cit*). That recognition is a growing certainty that culminates in the process of permanent ecstatic self-transcendence, known as "liberation," which is full enlightenment.

The enlightened being does not look for fulfillment in and through any role that "it" may temporarily animate, because it is already blissful and immortal. There is no fear of death, and therefore there is no need for the countless "vision quests" by which the unenlightened individual tries to affirm his or her own existence and to outwit the cosmic law of entropy. The enlightened being is of course aware that the body-mind, or psychosomatic organism, with which it happens to be mysteriously associated (at least from the perspective of unenlightenment) will inevitably grow old and die.

But this dreaded fate does not perplex or disturb the enlightened being, because "it" also knows that the same Consciousness-Identity remains forever, regardless of whether the body-mind or even the entire universe is annihilated. In enlightenment there is no illusion of proprietorship. To adapt E.F. Schumacher's well-known phrase: In the economy of enlightenment, *infinite is beautiful.*

In the *Upanishads* and later works of Vedanta, the transcendental Reality is often characterized as the eternal "witness." It is the ultimate watcher of the contents of consciousness, the fleeting states of mind, the ongoing swirl of sensations, emotions, thought fragments, hunches, insights, desires, attitudes, and so on. The late Mircea Eliade, perhaps our century's greatest historian of religion, observed:

> It is impossible . . . to disregard one of India's greatest discoveries: that of consciousness as witness, of consciousness freed from its psychophysiological structures and their temporal conditioning, the consciousness of the "liberated" man, of him, that is, who has succeeded in emancipating himself from temporality and thereafter knows the true, inexpressible freedom. [1]

The notion of the transcendental Witness was indeed an important conceptual innovation, which stood at the fountainhead of the entire ascetical tradition of Hinduism. And yet, it proved to be a double-edged sword. On one side, it cut through the conventional materialistic idealism that projects the empirical subject, or ego, into dimensions in which it has no place. Thus, it effectively undermined the archaic ideal of immortality in some post-mortem Elysium in the delightful company of the gods.

On the other side, however, it tended to lop off conventional life, which, it was thought, has nothing to do with the Witness. The Upanishadic procedure recommended for realizing the transcendental Self-Identity, beyond all roles, was to progressively disown everything that is generally considered to belong to normal human existence: family, social life, work, and, ultimately, the body-mind itself. *Neti neti*, "not thus, not thus," responded the Upanishadic sages when asked about the nature of the Self. The spiritual practitioner was expected to apply this wisdom to his or her everyday life, which was supposed to be simple and contemplative. The tradition of renunciation (*samnyasa, tyaga*) is characteristic of that attitude of negation.

Thus, the ideal of living liberation (*jivan-mukti*) was an important step in humanity's spiritual evolution. Yet, it was not a big enough stride. For, even though people could now dedicate themselves to attaining enlightenment in this lifetime, they still had a problematic relationship to embodiment. For them, the body-mind and the world at large were something to be left behind, at least emotionally. The key prescription was dissociation.

As a result, they did not escape entirely the pull of the earlier archaic notion of immortality. While immortality was no longer viewed as a goal in the hereafter, it still involved a form of death: The spiritual aspirant had to voluntarily withdraw from the world and his or her body-mind, until the glorious moment of illumination was reached. The adept had to die a metaphorical death, involving an inner deadening to the world. Later, upon Self-realization, he or she could return to the world and live in it but not of it—like the proverbial lotus floating on muddied water.

This tradition has become the style associated in our minds with India's spirituality. Indeed, it was the tradition that dominated both Hindu and Buddhist cultures for centuries. Seldom is it realized that it was not the ultimate flower of the spiritual heritage of India. For, the Hindu and also the Buddhist genius has recognized the limitation inherent in the concept and ideal of the transcendental Witness. This recognition was expressed in a total reappraisal of the physical dimension of existence—in the great and unfortunately muchmaligned spiritual movement of Tantrism.

At the heart of Tantrism is the equation *samsara* = *nirvana*, which means that the conditional world of space-time is coessential with the unconditional dimension of existence beyond the spatiotemporal world. To most people, this will mean as little as Einstein's famous formula $E = mc^2$. So, a brief explanation is in order. *Samsara* is the world of change, as we experience it through our senses. According to the Tantric adepts, that finite world is only the outermost aspect of an infinitely complex field. By yogic means, they are able to identify with the total cosmic field.

From the point of view of the unenlightened consciousness, that total field lies beyond the known and knowable world. But what the Tantric masters have discovered is that this field is all there is. Therefore, it does not *really* lie beyond the world of change. Rather, it *underlies* conditional existence, and in the last analysis is not different from it.

This has profound implications for our human condition, which the Tantric adepts realized. Thus, they came to regard the body, and bodily existence in general, as the "temple of the Divine." No longer was the body viewed as a "foul-smelling bag of skin," but embodiment was seen as a unique opportunity to realize its hidden potential—the potential of divinity. This new attitude is pithily expressed in the *Kula-Arnava-Tantra*, an important Hindu Tantric work, in the following way:

> Without the body, how can the [highest] human goal be realized? Therefore, having acquired a bodily abode, one should perform meritorious (*punya*) actions. (I.18)

> Among the 8,400,000 [types of] bodies of embodied beings, the knowledge of Reality cannot be acquired except through a human [body]. (I.14)

What the Tantric masters aspired to was to create a transubstantiated body, which they called "adamantine" (*vajra*) or "divine" (*daiva*)—a body not made of flesh but of immortal substance, of Light. Instead of regarding the body as a meat tube doomed to fall prey to sickness and death, they viewed it as a dwelling-place for the Divine, and as the cauldron for accomplishing spiritual perfection. For them, enlightenment was a whole-body event.

The embodiment of an enlightened master is only apparent. His or her body is really the Body of all, and therefore he or she can assume any form at will. The Tantric adept (*siddha*) possesses a transubstantiated body, which is endowed with the great paranormal powers (*siddhi*). Thus the spiritual adepts have throughout India's history been celebrated and feared as great thaumaturgists.

The magical element of Tantrism came to the fore in the tradition of "body-cultivation" (*kaya-sadhana*), notably the schools of *hatha-yoga*, which emerged in the tenth century A.D. Coming mostly from the illiterate social strata of Hindu society, the *hatha-yogins* often tended to misunderstand the body-positive teachings of Tantrism. Instead of realizing that the physical body cannot survive indefinitely, and that the immortal Tantric body is of a spiritual and not a material order, they went to great lengths to try to immortalize their mortal frames.

Thus, they invented an impressive range of techniques for controlling the bodily functions—from practices that effectively arrest breathing to methods of preventing seminal discharge. In *hatha-yoga*, at its coarsest, we have the ancient Vedic hope for immortality transferred to the physical level.

I have always defended *hatha-yoga* against scholarly prejudice, but it is nonetheless true that the ideal of bodily immortality is no more than a pipe dream that, moreover, can be dangerous to the dreamer. Of course, there may well be adepts with extraordinary lifespans. In fact, I have written an introduction to a biography of one of them, Tapasviji Maharaj, whose life is as well documented as we can expect in India's timeless culture.

We can learn from these exceptional ascetics—among other things—that they, like the rest of us, are destined to die in the end. No ideology and no technology can prevent this fate. Everything that is born must die. More precisely, everything that *experiences* itself to be born (i.e., the ego-self) must die. Hence the transcendental Self is traditionally said to be unborn (*aja*).

Our modern culture is apt to become fascinated with long-lived individuals like Tapasviji Maharaj or Shivapuri Baba, and with the ideal of physical immortality. The emergent medical discipline of genetic engineering is our contemporary secular answer to the ancient method of *kaya-kalpa* ("body-fashioning"), a naturopathic way of rejuvenating the body through prolonged fasting, meditation, and special herbal remedies. For what is it that genetic engineers ultimately hope to accomplish, if not the extension of life?

However, while genetic engineering may succeed in adding years and perhaps even well-being to our lives, it cannot presolve the spiritual lessons that each person must learn for himself or herself. And those lessons will be in the future, as they are now, bound up with the inescapable fact that physical existence is finite, very finite, and that to give human life deep and lasting meaning, we must include in its purview the glorious dimension of what the sages and mystics of India have anciently called "Being-Consciousness-Bliss."

We are today in the thick of a sweeping cultural transition. As Friedrich Nietzsche boldly declared a century ago, the parental Creator-God of our forebears has died for most of us. We can no longer believe in paradise and the resurrection of the flesh. But we are still mourning this loss, and are certainly perplexed. Some of us have become sensitive to a new possibility—a possibility long realized on Indian soil, namely that Reality is immanent *and* transcendental, and that we can discover this truth existentially and not merely intellectually, precisely because It *is* us.

Of course, the rational mind wonders at all of this. This is how it should be, for doubt is the province of reason. But then there is also the heart, which rejoices at such a possibility. Together, head and heart will aid our spiritual quest. We can feel free to listen to the whispers of immortality.

NOTE

1. M. Eliade, *Yoga: Immortality and Freedom* (Princeton, NJ: Princeton University, 1973), p. xx.

26

LIVING IN THE DARK AGE (KALI-YUGA)

The idea that we live either at the brink of Armageddon or at the dawn of a new golden age is becoming ever more prominent even as we approach the end of the second millennium A.D. Some critics have acidly observed that people throughout the ages have always believed they were living in particularly crucial times. There is some truth to this criticism, because human history is indeed continuously decisive, for in humanity's march through time every step determines the future of our species. But only the cynic would sneer at the idea that some steps, some historical periods, are more decisive than others—not only in the shaping of a particular race or nation, but for humanity as a whole.

Possibly one such decisive historical threshold was what the German philosopher and psychiatrist Karl Jaspers styled the "axial age"—the period between 800–500 B.C. when "thought turned back upon thought": the epoch of Confucius, Lao Tzu, Buddha, Zoroaster, Heraclitus, Plato, and Socrates.

In the West, this development gradually led to what can only be described as the enthronement and autarchy of cold reason and the consequent suppression of nonrational modes of consciousness. As many contemporary thinkers have shown, this inflation of *ratio* lies at the root of today's moral and spiritual bankruptcy, and its disastrous effects can be witnessed all around us (and in us, if we care to look).

What is perhaps most disheartening is that this lopsided orientation to life is now being thrust upon the "underdeveloped" world, which merely magnifies the existing threat to our planet's ecology and to the survival of countless life forms, not least our own human species.

When we take stock of the folly of humankind we begin to realize the extent of the global problems induced, in the last analysis, by hypertrophied reason. We may also be impressed with the traditional Hindu explanation of the particular spirit of our era. For, according to the computations of the Hindu pundits, we are well into the "dawn phase" of the *kali-yuga*, or "dark age."

Like so many premodern mythologies, Hinduism views the evolution of humanity as a cyclical process of progressive moral degeneration from an original state of purity and spiritual wholeness. The Sanskrit sources distinguish four stages in this drama:

1. *Krita-yuga*, also called *satya-yuga*, the golden age of harmony and truth (*satya*);

2. *treta-yuga*, lit., the "age of the thrice(-lucky)";

3. *dvapara-yuga*, lit., the "age of the twice(-lucky)";

4. *kali-yuga*, lit., the "dark age."

This intriguing doctrine was elaborated in the late pre-Christian centuries, perhaps around the same time that the founding fathers of our Western civilization, the philosophers of Greece, Ionia, and Italy, started to express the new mode of consciousness.

The strange-sounding designations for these four epochs (*yuga*) are explained by the fact that they were adopted from the earlier Vedic tradition, where they stood for certain throws of dice—*krita* being the luckiest and *kali* being the unlucky throw. It is not clear how these gambling terms came to acquire their new meaning, but why they did can be gleaned from the respective duration postulated for each world age. This is best conveyed in tabular form:

	DIVINE YEARS	HUMAN YEARS
Krita-yuga-samdhya (Morning Twilight Phase)	400	144,000
Krita-yuga	4,000	1,440,000
Krita-yuga-samdhya-amsha (Evening Twilight Phase)	400	144,000
Treta-yuga-samdhya (Morning Twilight Phase)	300	108,000
Treta-yuga	3,000	1,080,000
Treta-yuga-samdhya-amsha (Evening Twilight Phase)	300	108,000

	DIVINE YEARS	HUMAN YEARS
Dvapara-yuga-samdhya (Morning Twilight Phase)	200	72,000
Dvapara-yuga	2,000	720,000
Dvapara-yuga-samdhya-amsha (Evening Twilight Phase)	200	72,000
Kali-yuga-samdhya (Morning Twilight Phase)	100	36,000
Kali-yuga	1,000	360,000
Kali-yuga-samdhya-amsha (Evening Twilight Phase)	100	36,000
	12,000 =	4,320,000

From the above tabulation we can see that while the *krita-yuga* comes in fours, the *treta-yuga* is based on a computation of threes and the *dvapara-yuga* of twos. The world ages are thus considered progressively less auspicious.

The computation further indicates that we are dealing here with "divine years" which, when translated into human terms, yield immense spans of time. But Hindu chronology does not stop there. The four world ages are collectively known as a *maha-yuga* or "great age," and it is thought that two thousand of these supercycles form but a single dawn and night (called *kalpa*) in the life of the Creator (God Brahma). His life-span extends over a "century," that is, a period of 311,040,000,000,000 human years.

At the demise of the Creator, the whole manifest universe becomes dissolved. After an immeasurable period, the process is reversed and the whole cycle of space-time existence starts all over again. A truly awesome vision! It leaves no doubt about the utter insignificance of the human race, never mind the individual.

Only the liberated being has cause for humor, for the *jivan-mukta* stands well clear of this cosmic *perpetuum mobile*. His or her dissolution is not merely a temporary respite from the whirling wheel of existence, but it amounts to a permanent establishment in the transcendental condition of Being-Consciousness-Bliss. This unsurpassable attainment is called "absolute dissolution" (*atyantika-pralaya*) and is distinct from both *pralaya* and *maha-pralaya*.

Where do we of today stand in this immense time game? As I have mentioned already, we find ourselves in the opening phase

of the last of the four world ages. According to the Hindu mythochronologers, the present *kali-yuga* (morning twilight phase)
commenced on February 18, 3102 B.C. This date marks the memo-
rable battle on the *kuru-kshetra*, the great war recorded in the
Mahabharata epic. Some authorities, however, place the beginning
slightly later to commemorate the ascension of the incarnate God
Krishna, thirty-six years after the Bharata war. There are several
more views, however, that converge on roughly the same century.
But these differences are of marginal significance only.

What is of interest, however, is the characterization of the *yugas*
in general and of the *kali-yuga* in particular. We find that the descriptions are remarkably uniform in the various scriptures dealing
with the world ages, such as the *Smriti* (ritual texts), the *Mahabharata* epic, the *Puranas* (popular encyclopedias), and also the
works on astronomy. The following is a quotation from the
Mahabharata which describes our present era and the immediately
preceding *yuga*, revealing a progressive deterioration of humanity's
moral fiber.

> Again, in the *dvapara-yuga* the moral order (*dharma*) exists [only]
> half. [God] Vishnu becomes yellow, and the *Veda* is now four-fold
> [i.e., the original wisdom is split into the four Vedic hymnodies].
>
> Thence, some [adhere to] four *Vedas*, others to three *Vedas*, or two
> *Vedas*, or a single *Veda*, while yet others have no hymns [at all].
>
> Thus, owing to the broken traditions, rites become manifold and
> creatures, fond of austerities and almsgiving, become *rajas*-
> motivated.[1]
>
> Due to ignorance about the single *Veda*, the *Vedas* become multiple
> and because of the collapse of truth, few adhere to truthfulness.
>
> Many diseases appear for those who have fallen from truth, and
> there are desires and disasters caused by fate. Afflicted by these,
> [some] men perform very severe austerities; others, filled with
> [worldly] desires or desiring heaven, conduct sacrifices.
>
> Thus with the onset of the *dvapara*, creatures perish through their
> lawlessness. In the *kali-yuga*, O Kaunteya, the moral order
> (*dharma*) exists by one quarter only.

With the onset of this *tamas*-motivated Age, Keshava [i.e., God Vishnu] becomes black (*krishna*).[2] The Vedic ways-of-life end, and so do the moral order, sacrifice, and rites.

Plagues, disease, sloth, blemishes such as anger, as well as calamities, sickness, and afflictions prevail.

In the course of the *yugas*, the moral order diminishes increasingly. With the diminution of the moral order, the people (*loka*) diminish.

This description of the *kali-yuga* is not as daunting as it is in some other scriptures. But the message is clear enough: Ours is a sinister age. What thinking person would not agree? Can we not, by now, fill a whole library with tales of human foolishness, of humanity's thoughtless interference with the life-world and its almost unbelievable lack of concern for fellow beings, both human and nonhuman?

Is there, then, no hope for humankind? Is historian Oswald Spengler's dark prophecy of the decline of the West (and with it, also of the East) coming true?[3] Or are there, today, forces at work that countermand the *Zeitgeist,* the spirit of the age? This latter is indeed so. It could not be otherwise. Or else our species would have perished long ago, right at the outset of the *kali-yuga.*

The *kali-yuga*, then, does not signal *total* spiritual darkness or inevitable doom. Inverting a popular maxim, one can perhaps say that where there is shadow there is also light. The present dark age is, here and there, pierced by shafts of light. It is not without its benign counterbalancing influences.

According to the Hindu tradition, shortly before the dawn of the *kali-yuga*, on the eve of one of the fiercest wars fought in antiquity, the Divine critically intervened in human affairs. It revealed itself in the form of the God-man Krishna, who acted as a charioteer on the side of Prince Arjuna's military force. Just before the first battle between the two mighty armies, representing good and evil respectively, Lord Krishna instructed the virtuous prince in spiritual matters.

Krishna's message is of particular interest not least because it is a teaching that was framed in response to an imminent "holocaust"—the kind of disastrous human action that is typical of the *kali-yuga.* It requires no special imaginative skills to perceive the parallel between the fateful situation faced by Prince Arjuna and our present-day crisis.

At that time—just as today—the evil machinations of a few power-hungry individuals with no regard for the larger good had created an intolerable situation demanding to be redressed. As is so often true, circumstances and human will conspired that this restoration of law and order should be accomplished by an all-out military confrontation.

Prince Arjuna, though born into the warrior estate, was at heart a peace-loving man. When the two colossal armies lined up on opposite sides, he began to have serious doubts about his task. It was not so much personal fear of death that swayed his heart but, rather, acute moral qualms. Has anyone the right, he wondered, to use force in order to promote the larger good? His dilemma was greatly aggravated by the fact that among those whom he was supposed to fight—maim and possibly kill—were kinsmen and revered teachers.

Arjuna's duty as a warrior was clear enough; he had to fight. But the moment he contemplated the larger implications of this action, he was terrified to abide by his decision to reconquer his lost kingdom. Arjuna's attitude is typical of human life itself. We are all the time engaged in decision-making or in decision-avoidance. The more consciously we live, the more we realize that life is really an incessant stream of potential decisions.

Arjuna, as we know, did fight his war and also emerged victorious. But *first* he had to learn an important spiritual lesson. Lord Krishna, who acted as his charioteer, convinced the prince that his whole confusion was the result of a faulty perspective. The God-man demonstrated to the prince that the problem that caused him such anxiety was a problem conjured up by the ego. It had no existence apart from the ego. The divine teacher made Arjuna understand that we can never transcend our circumstances merely by closing our eyes, by avoiding action, by dropping out. Even avoidance is an action, which will have its inevitable repercussions since avoidance is rooted in the ego.

What Lord Krishna recommended instead was a cognitive shift, a new view of the whole matter: away from the delimiting, anxious ego and toward the boundless Self. All action must be sacrifice, he explained. We must not hold on to any conventional ego-derived schemas. Only when we abandon the delusion that we, as ego-personalities, are the ultimate initiators of actions can we have knowledge of what is truly right and good. That is to say, when we discover the "witness," the Self, we realize that life unfolds spontaneously and mysteriously, and that the ego is merely one of the countless forms arising within the flux of life.

For the Hindu authorities, the general deterioration of spirituality and the decline of humanity's psychological health in no way precludes the possibility of spiritual aspiration and success. It is nowhere denied that contemporary humanity, feeble as it may be in comparison to its ancestors, can swim against the stream. On the contrary, all spiritual teachings affirm that we must do our utmost to cultivate spiritual values in the midst of the great darkness surrounding us.

In fact, the tradition of Tantrism, which emerged in the early post-Christian centuries, purports to be a spiritual discipline specifically for the dark age. It is clearly based on the belief that we can and must improve our spiritual destiny. Whatever the age, we are inherently capable of transcending the particular circumstances of our time. However dense the *kali-yuga* may become, human beings will always be able to conjure up within themselves the characteristics of the golden age, the *satya-yuga*, marked by freedom, joy, and love.

This is so because whatever degree of moral corruption may befall us, in our essence we are neither space-bound nor time-dependent. Therefore, by an inward act, we can always remove ourselves from the values and attitudes of our particular epoch or culture and cultivate those values and attitudes that reflect the purer characteristics of the *dvapara-*, the *treta-*, or even the *satya-yuga*.

Yet, it appears, exceedingly few people today exercise their radical freedom to choose higher values and forms of life surpassing the conditions of the dark age. As we have learned from the above-quoted passage from the *Mahabharata* epic, lethargy is a function of our time, which is ruled by *tamas*, or the principle of inertia.

The general pessimism of the Hindu mythochronologers is not shared by many Western enthusiasts of astrology. They celebrate the passage of the equinoxes through the constellation of Aquarius, in

March 1948, as ushering in a new age in which humankind will come to fulfill its earthly destiny.

The symbol of this new age is the Water Bearer who, with the Water of Immortality contained in a pitcher, irrigates and thus fertilizes Nature. This new era has been explained as coinciding with the realization of true humanity on earth: the unification of humankind through science and technology on one hand, and through the biological-spiritual ideal of "friendship" on the other. There are high hopes and expectations in new age circles.

This optimism has given rise both to a new mythology that tends toward the baroque and to a number of rather eccentric cults. There are, however, also more serious manifestations of new age thought, and these are slowly gaining influence in the larger society. They coexist side by side with the destructive forces of our age, which extend from rampant consumerism, scientific materialism, and technocratic ideology to religious fundamentalism, racism, and militarism.

One of the more sober efforts to articulate the *Zeitgeist* is found in the monumental study by the Swiss cultural philosopher Jean Gebser (1905–1973). In his work *The Ever-Present Origin*, he presented a large body of evidence that something new is indeed trying to crystallize in our midst.[4] In his penetrating analysis of the history of human consciousness, Gebser arrived at the startling conclusion that the present global crisis is but the outer reverberation of a drastic "mutation" of consciousness, the transformation of the dualistic-rational mode of world perception into what he calls the "integral" structure of consciousness.

After a most careful scrutiny of the sciences, music, architecture, painting, and—with particular illumination—language itself, Gebser discovered a host of significant signposts pointing out the direction that this emergent consciousness might take if we but nurture it. Whatever else it might bring about, it will first and foremost help us to actualize *ego-transcendence*. Gebser felt that without this realization humanity cannot possibly hope to master the problems that lie ahead.

It is reassuring that Gebser's general thesis, first conceived in

1932, has independently been voiced by at least two other intellectual giants—the Hindu philosopher-sage Sri Aurobindo and the
French priest and paleontologist Pierre Teilhard de Chardin.
Whereas Sri Aurobindo spoke of the descent of the "Supermind,"
Teilhard de Chardin invented the concept of the "*Omega* point," the
spiritual evolutionary destiny of humanity. [5] During the past two decades, numerous other thinkers have formulated their own version
of what is happening today. I have discussed a cross-section of their
work in my book *Structures of Consciousness.* [6] Many agree that, our
era's perils notwithstanding, we are witnessing a potent tendency
toward a more benign future.

This is an encouraging insight or belief. And what is more encouraging still is the fact that these scholars are now part of a small
but increasingly vociferous minority. Should the spiritual wasteland
become arable once again? Or are these hopeful signs only so many
will-o'-the-wisps? Is the Aquarian Age only a sub-cycle within the
larger cycle of the *kali-yuga,* or is the Hindu view simply in error?

Leaving aside for the moment certain occult reinterpretations of the
yugas (which are drastically shortened to suit astrological purposes), a
number of the *Puranas* contain a puzzling but undoubtedly significant
statement. According to these Sanskrit scriptures, the whole bold
structure of the *yuga* theory applies only to Bharatavarsha, that is, India! Admittedly, this smacks of a critical afterthought by editors or
scribes who have come into contact with non-Indian chronologies and
obviously felt the need to justify their own native tradition. But their
qualification is nonetheless fascinating.

Whatever the truth about the Hindu model of world ages may be,
in determining our individual response to life we can rely neither on
the *yuga* theory nor on any of the contending new age explanations
of the spirit of our times. Rather, we must realize that, as individuals
and to some extent as a group, we determine our own future. We
can embody either the dark actualities of our age or its luminous
potential. We can help shape gloom and doom or increase the light
in the world. The choice is always ours.

NOTES

1. The Sanskrit term *rajas* stands for the dynamic quality in Nature, which is traditionally used to apply to both external and psychological manifestations.

2. The Sanskrit word *tamas* denotes "inertia," one of the three principal forces of Nature, the other two being *rajas* (the principle of dynamism) and *sattva* (the principle of lucidity). In the golden age, the *sattva* principle was overwhelmingly prevalent. It was increasingly undermined by the other two principles in subsequent world ages.

3. See O. Spengler, *Der Untergang des Abendlandes* (Munich: Beck, 1963).

4. See J. Gebser, *The Ever-Present Origin* (Athens: Ohio University Press, 1986).

5. See, e.g., Sri Aurobindo, *The Life Divine* (Pondicherry, India: Sri Aurobindo Ashram, 1977), 2 vols. See also, e.g., P. Teilhard de Chardin, *The Future of Man* (London: Collins, 1964).

6. See G. Feuerstein, *Structures of Consciousness: The Genius of Jean Gebser—An Introduction and Critique* (Lower Lake, CA: Integral Publishing, 1987).

RECOMMENDED READING

This short bibliography is in addition to the reading lists provided at the end of essays 4 and 5 and the works mentioned in the other essays of the present volume.

Aivanhov, Mikhael. *The Yoga of Nutrition.* Frejus, France: Prosveta, 1982.

_____. *Toward a Solar Civilisation.* Frejus, France: Prosveta, 1982.

Anand, Margo. *The Art of Sexual Ecstasy: The Path of Sacred Sexuality for Western Lovers.* Los Angeles: J.P. Tarcher, 1990.

Brunton, Paul. *The Notebooks of Paul Brunton.* Burdett, NY: Larson Publications, 1984–1988. Vols. 1–16.

Eliade, Mircea. *Patanjali and Yoga.* New York: Schocken Books, 1976.

Feuerstein, Georg. *Yoga: The Technology of Ecstasy.* Los Angeles: J.P. Tarcher, 1989.

_____. *Encyclopedic Dictionary of Yoga.* New York: Paragon House, 1990.

_____. *Enlightened Sexuality: Essays on Body-Positive Spirituality.* Freedom, CA: Crossing Press, 1989.

King, Francis. *Tantra: The Way of Action.* Rochester, VT: Destiny Books, 1990.

Laski, Marghanita. *Ecstasy in Secular and Religious Experiences.* Los Angeles: J.P. Tarcher, 1990.

Motoyama, Hiroshi. *Toward a Superconsciousness: Meditational Theory and Practice.* Berkeley, CA: Asian Humanities Press, 1990.

Raju, P.T. *Structural Depths of Indian Thought.* New York: SUNY Press, 1985.

Swami Sivananda Radha. *Hatha Yoga: The Hidden Language.* Porthill, ID: Timeless Books, 1987.

Varenne, Jean. *Yoga and the Hindu Tradition*. Chicago, IL: University of Chicago Press, 1976.

Walsh, Roger. *The Spirit of Shamanism*. Los Angeles: J.P. Tarcher, 1990.

White, John, ed. *Kundalini: Evolution and Enlightenment*. New York: Paragon House, 1990.

_____, ed. *What is Enlightenment? Exploring the Goal of the Spiritual Path*. Los Angeles: J.P. Tarcher, 1985.

INDEX